MEET
Your
BODY

of related interest

Bagua Daoyin
A Unique Branch of Daoist Learning, A Secret Skill of the Palace
He Jinghan
Translated by David Alexander
ISBN 978 1 84819 009 2

You Are How You Move
Experiential Chi Kung
Ged Sumner
ISBN 978 1 84819 014 6

Integrated Yoga
Yoga with a Sensory Integrative Approach
Nicole Cuomo
ISBN 978 1 84310 862 7

MEET
Your
BODY

CORE BODYWORK
AND ROLFING
TOOLS TO RELEASE
BODYMINDCORE
TRAUMA

Noah Karrasch

Illustrated by Lovella Lindsey Norrell

Foreword by Ralph Harvey, MD

SINGING
DRAGON

London and Philadelphia

First published in 2009
by Singing Dragon
An imprint of Jessica Kingsley Publishers
116 Pentonville Road
London N1 9JB, UK
and
400 Market Street, Suite 400
Philadelphia, PA 19106, USA

www.singing-dragon.com

Library of Congress Cataloging in Publication Data
Karrasch, Noah.
Meet your body : a Rolfer's guide to releasing bodymindcore trauma / Noah Karrasch ;
illustrated by Lovella Lindsey.
p. cm.
ISBN 978-1-84819-016-0 (pb : alk. paper) 1. Rolfing. I. Title.
RC489.R64K37 2009
615.8'22--dc22
2008041281
British Library Cataloguing in Publication Data
A CIP catalogue record for this book is available from the British Library

ISBN 978 1 84819 016 0
eISBN 978 0 85701 000 1

Printed and bound in Great Britain

*This book is dedicated to all my teachers:
my clients, my family, my friends, my colleagues,
and most especially my partner Gloria, the teacher who
has helped me acknowledge and unwind deep layers of
fear, anxiety, elation and joy.
Blessings to you all.*

*To all who have gone before: I hope I've shined a
different light on the path we're all pursuing.*

ACKNOWLEDGMENTS

Emmett Hutchins, Peter Melchior, Louis Schultz, and Stacey Mills for their gentle nudges in the right direction.

Colleagues past and present on both sides of the Atlantic, especially Greg and Jennifer Peterson, Drew Clark, Ibby Garvey, Juliet Mee, Frank Lack, Gilli Hanna, Monica Stefaniuk, Michael Kauffman, Gillian Hamer, Chris Salvary, Susan Findlay, Elizabeth Heren, and Bev Breeze.

Ida P. Rolf, Jim Oschmann, Leon Chaitow, and Tom Myers for their groundbreaking development of myofascial bodywork.

Dr. Ralph Harvey, many times great descendant of Dr. William Harvey, discoverer of the circulatory system. We're continuing the work, Ralph.

Dr. Chris Link for advice, support, questions, and trust.

Jessica Kingsley for her faith in me and my topic.

All my students, friends, and clients who have taught me so much.

George Galanes, who taught me that every encounter is a chance for a wonderful experience.

My daughter Molly for many faithful years as a parenting novice's guineapig.

CONTENTS

FOREWORD

By Ralph Harvey, MD

As a physician, I see many complaints and problems that patients bring to us that don't fit into the narrow boxes we learned in medical school. The concepts in this book are not commonly taught in medical school, but they are crucial to an understanding of how our bodies actually work, and how we can take ourselves from hurt, through healing, towards optimal health.

Often, the place a patient experiences pain is not the source of the pain, or dysfunction. For example: a patient came in complaining of severe right knee pain. As he worked with a physical therapist, it became evident that his core dysfunction was in his hip. He favored his right hip as he walked, and placed extra stress on his knee. The knee hurt, but healing was found in the hip, low back, and ultimately, addressing how the entire back and legs were functioning.

I often tell my patients that we have four sides: Physical, Emotional, Intellectual, and Spiritual. Nothing affects just one side. Any event will have an impact on all four sides of our being. For example, take a physical illness like the flu. When you have a temperature of 104 degrees, every bone and every muscle in the body aches. It is a physical illness, but intellectually, is this a time to make a detailed financial analysis? NO! Is it a time for a deep emotional discussion with a loved one? NO! Spiritually, few people can get past "Oh God, Help!" What we call a *physical* illness affects all aspects of our being.

Noah's bodymindcore focuses primarily on the physical connections of the body, but he incorporates and includes the entire person—however we choose to describe ourselves. His concept of twenty-one hinges in the body presents a practical and functional approach to healing and health.

Where will *Meet Your Body* fit into my primary care practice? I think it will become a primary resource for those people who are serious about actively pursuing their own health and healing. It is not for the person wanting a quick, or easy, fix; or a magic pill or magic stretch that will fix everything. But I see his work as central to a practical approach to healing, and a path towards optimal health.

I have known about Rolfing since 1970, and went through my first Rolfing series around 1971. I have personally known profound physical healing through Rolfing. I've known Noah for about twenty years, as a Rolfer, friend, and brother-in-law. He is a gifted Rolfer, body worker, and teacher.

Ralph Harvey
MD Diplomate, ABFM, Associate Professor, Department
of Family Medicine, Michigan State University—College of
Human Medicine

PROLOGUE

I've been a practicing bodyworker for twenty-three years and have taught bodywork skills for the past fifteen of them. In that time I've seen lots of distressed bodies and spirits, and worked with interesting conditions, including some in my own body. My personal major crisis came over twenty years ago when I was in a small plane that crash-landed, breaking my spine and causing me to have surgery to clean, fuse, and stabilize it. Most friends and students believe I've rehabilitated myself quite well.

WHAT I DO, WHAT I SEE

A word about my credentials: I studied at the Rolf Institute from 1984–86, after having read Ida Rolf's book *Ida Rolf Talks About Rolfing and Physical Reality* (Rosemary Feitis, 1978, Rochester, VT: Healing Arts Press). As I read her words, I knew she was speaking common sense, directly to me. I abandoned a successful music career to pursue certification at the Institute. I've never looked back. Currently I still practice Rolfing but lean toward my own style of work, which I've named CORE Bodywork. The acronym CORE stands for: Coax Order, Restore Ease. I believe it's my challenge to identify stuck places in the connective tissue network of my clients, and invite them to release old trauma held in this network. It's satisfying work; yet I'm still interested in helping more people come to the realization that tension is meant to be released.

I've begun to see generalities and similarities in all bodies and have decided it's time to share my ideas with a larger circle beyond the clients and students I now serve. Recently I began writing a student textbook. As I finished, I realized that book was too complex for my clients—it was written to challenge a bodyworker who already had specialized learning and skills. There were just too many technical terms and ideas to confuse an inquisitive person who's interested in getting to know and use their own body better.

That's where this book comes into play. I've come upon a way to present important information that I believe *any body*, no matter its level of body knowledge and mechanics, could benefit from and use to enhance its own being and doing. I'm eager to share with you these ideas to help you get to know your body and turn around your life.

DIS-EASE IS THE SLOWDOWN OF ENERGY

I believe there's only one dis-ease, and it's the slowdown of energy. Too many of us hold onto old patterns of tension because we don't know how to get beyond them. I hope to challenge you to look at your patterns and discern which are serving you positively and which serve you negatively. You can choose to sort these behaviors and reprogram yourself to create more positive patterns in your life and your world. I'll tell you up front: I'm going to ask you to slow down and really get to know your body intimately.

HINGES IN OUR BODY: CLEAN THEM, REALIGN THEM

This book is based on a model that each of our bodies is composed of many important hinges; if we can just "oil" and free these hinges so that energy moves through them, our bodymindcore will be open and receptive to good things moving through our lives and our worlds. In each chapter we'll work with a specific hinge. While you may want to jump right to the chapter where you find problems in your own body (for example, the knees), know that the goal of the book is to get you to think in terms of lengthening the body, pulling all the hinges away from each other, and adding resiliency, strength and stretch to each hinge *and* the entire being. So, don't get focused on only your "bad" hinges; remember to work with them all. Don't just meet your problem hinge; meet its neighbors too.

The hinges I'd like you to know more fully are: big toes, ankles, knees, hips, lumbosacral or sacred, stomach, heart, arms, shoulders, elbows, wrists, fingers and head. Of course, we can argue there are many "extra" hinges: the spine alone has twenty-six that I've reduced to my five most important ones. We'll begin at the ground and work our way up through the body, because our foundation is on the ground. Any work that happens above must be based on the way our feet and legs relate to the ground.

I'm getting more convinced that we simply need to

learn to isolate and feel these hinges, stretch them, and then connect and stretch them to the hinges farther up and down the lines of holding we all carry in our bodies. It's my goal to help you learn how to stretch and oil your own hinges.

BODYMINDCORE

A word about bodymindcore is appropriate here. To my knowledge, I coined this term to explain how we really can't separate our emotions from our bodies or vice versa—some of us have psychosomatic illnesses in our heads, caused by our emotions. Others have somatopsychic illness—our bodies hurt so badly they affect our minds. Both of these illnesses tighten and shorten our cores as we try to protect the essence of who we are. If I can help you unwind your bodymindcore—whether from the body, from the emotions, or from any starting point we find— I'm assisting you in freeing and knowing your essence, your core experience, your being and your doing. This is my goal.

Each chapter addresses a particular hinge physically as well as sharing ideas about its emotional component. We'll ask what you can do for yourself to operate a hinge more efficiently so as to invite the entire being to open. It's holy work I'm inviting you to undertake. You're worth it! I'm less interested in teaching you routines, and more interested in teaching you to think and act in new ways that allow you to open all your hinges and move through them happily. Let's go to work!

THE BIG TOE HINGE

THE OLD SAYINGS MAKE SENSE

Think about the old phrases relating to our bodies that we've all heard and used: He's a pain in the neck (or lower). He made me sick to my stomach and I'm tied in knots. She makes me weak in the knees. I feel the weight of the world on my shoulders. I've got my head in the clouds and my feet on the ground. I'll dig in my heels and survive. This work keeps me on my toes.

All these sayings, based on body parts, make perfect sense. We do get our stomachs tied in knots when we find we have trouble expressing ourselves. We do carry the weight of the world on our shoulders when we believe we're in charge of our small section of the universe. We dig in our heels to survive, and we work to stay on our toes. The trouble is, we often work too hard to stay on our toes, or we surrender and lose them; we've forgotten how to find joyful "neutral".

I'd like you to realize that you're very possibly not fully living in your toe hinges, especially the big toe's hinges. *I believe that many of us on the planet at this time would rather not be here.* Some of us don't feel safe in life, so we tiptoe on eggshells, or hot coals, or broken glass as we walk through it. Some seem to me to be "de-feet-ed". We've surrendered so far into the ground that we have absolutely no integrity left in the tissues above our tired, collapsed feet. The lucky third group has joy in every step as their feet carry them forward. I'd like to help everyone see how they might join this latter group.

Foot placement strongly relates to an art many of us know well: the art of self sabotage. How grounded are we? How resilient is our contact to the earth? Do we enjoy our time on the planet, or do we continue to walk as if the earth might betray us at the next step, and so set ourselves up for failure? Perhaps I tiptoe through life, or perhaps I collapse in "de-feet". Yet when I feel good about myself, joyfully walk through life, and see every step as an exciting move into a glorious future, I live in a far different world. I expect good things to happen to me, and they do.

THE BALANCE POINTS OF THE FOOT

For years I've been suggesting to clients and students that we need to put our weight equally between four points on each foot. Those points are the ball of the great toe (1), ball of the outer toe (2), inner heel (3) and outer heel (4). I've even asked clients to add two more points to this map: the inside (5) and outside (6) middle or transverse arch, those points halfway down the foot inside and outside.

Too many of us put most of our weight in the heels of both feet and on the outer arch line so that our weight pulls away from the inner arch (2, 4, 6). Flat-footed people may put more weight on their inner arch—the defeated,

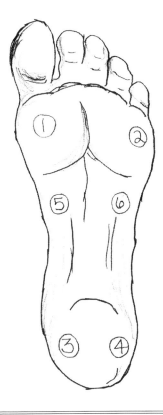

*Figure 1.1 Equal balance between
six different points of the footbed*

who have lost their toe hinge. Some people actually tiptoe through life and rarely let their heels touch the ground at all (1, 2). Their hinge never gets totally used. I'd like to encourage you to find a new stance, based on toes that hinge easily and usefully.

Take a moment to examine *your* stance. Remember my six points of connection: Which points touch the ground most for you? Are you in your inner arches, or your outer ones? Does one foot carry more weight than the other?

Experiment with changing that pattern: if you stand primarily in the right foot, transfer more weight to the left. If you're in your heels and outer arches, move to the toes and inner arches. Next, look at the direction of your feet. Does one or do both big toes point outside, or are your feet on straight? Point both feet straight ahead and put them six to eight inches apart. Many people feel pigeon-toed by just trying to get their feet under them correctly. Align your feet, keeping equal weight in both feet and legs. Practice staying there.

Why do most of us have such crooked stances? Possibilities are endless. A stance could have developed from something as simple as an injured ankle, a broken bone in a foot or leg, or even a hip or shoulder injury. It could be from crossing legs in one direction all the time, or having driven a car too much. It could relate to feeling closer to one parent, thereby putting weight in the side that usually represents father (right) or mother (left) influence. Speculating on *why* any of us has created our particular pattern, while fascinating, isn't our goal. *Our goal is to get us out of the pattern of unbalanced weight distribution, and to learn to spring from the toe hinge, so that we can connect with and exercise the deep line of the body through that hinge.*

CHECK YOUR ALIGNMENT

After you've decided where your feet belong, check your knees. Did they change direction when your feet realigned? Putting feet on straight may make one or both knees feel they're turning in; or that they're now weak or painful. This isn't wrong, it just is. Observe it. I tell clients their feet are the tires on their vehicle and their knees are the headlights. What do your tracks look like? Are you wearing out one or both tires? Are your knees lighting your path, or spreading their light somewhere off to a side? The goal is good *tracking*—the feet and the knees all pointing straight ahead. Try a knee bend where both knees and feet track straight ahead. How strange does that feel to you?

Stacey Mills was one of my instructors at the Rolf Institute. She'd come to Rolfing from the psychology community, so she often evaluated and correlated body parts to emotional situations. She told me that in thirty years of Rolfing clients, she'd found only two people who came to their first session with their feet fitting straight ahead in a truly structurally efficient pattern. Both were Catholic priests who'd known from an early age they wanted to be priests *and had felt totally supported* by their families in that calling.

Her observation suggests that the clearer we are in life direction, the more efficient the direction of our feet, legs and body will be. When we know where we're going, our feet and legs happily take us there! When we sabotage ourselves with every step, it takes much longer to get where we're going!

Examine a favorite pair of shoes you've had for a while. Many of us see one or both heels are worn more on the outside. Can you see how such a wear pattern not only tells you you're walking incorrectly, but that continuing to wear these old shoes is further ingraining an unhealthy walking and standing pattern in you? Can you see why it's important to get rid of old shoes with unhealthy wear patterns? How can you be in your toes if your shoes set you back on your heels?

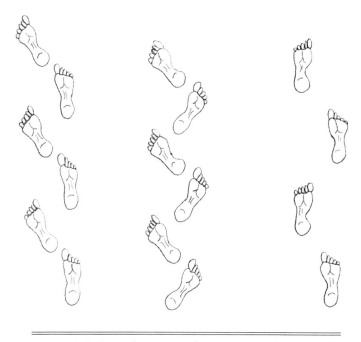

Figure 1.2 Foot alignment changes everything above

I've spent many dollars in the past few years on more and better shoes, and I've come to the realization that I need better legs, not better shoes. As a result of my wreck years ago that badly damaged my spine, my legs lost tone. My fused spine doesn't allow much spinal undulation or wave that would keep the legs resilient. I'm careful about what shoes I wear; I'm also becoming more interested in getting my feet and legs to energize and exercise. When I use my toe hinges regularly, I have far fewer problems through my entire body.

THE SECRET BEHIND THE BIG TOE

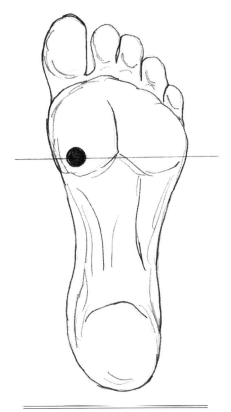

*Figure 1.3 A new balance point
for the body's weight*

Lately I've been concentrating on allowing weight to move mainly through one point, located right behind the big toe, just in front of where the big toe begins to join the inner arch of the foot. If we could truly learn to put our weight here and spring from this spot in our standing and walking, 80 percent of the health challenges we experience could go away. This is the spot I think of when I want to change someone's world. *If we can create a horizontal big toe hinge through this spot, our entire body will profit.*

Experiment with the idea you're on a diving board. Be ready to spring off that board. Rock back and forth— let yourself be too heavy in the heels, now too light in the toes. Make smaller and smaller adjustments until you find yourself just *slightly* in your big toes, slightly ready to jump. Can you feel movement and awareness through the feet and up the back of the calf? You may experience pain or burning, even cramping. Meet your calf muscles! Realize your legs need to liven up. Can you imagine how stretching and pumping deep calf muscles could ease varicose veins, knee problems, back pain, and much more? The movement of muscles asks your body to re-oil its toe hinges and stretch this shock absorber muscle in a way that supports everything above.

This hinge behind the big toe is the bottom of the deep line of the entire body and the basis of all succeeding chapters. There's a hidden muscle in your leg running from the spot behind the toe, under and behind the inside ankle bone, and all the way up the back of the leg, anchored deeply behind the two leg bones. It's called *tibialis posterior* (back of the tibia). If you can learn to find your big toe hinge spot, stand in it and walk from it with resiliency, you're well on the way to losing weight, getting rid of back pain, clearing plantar fasciitis, and feeling at ease in your body, because *you're learning to stretch this too-tight muscle.*

If you watch people walking, you'll see different hinges have been lost. Defeated people appear to shuffle through life without energy. They don't pick up their legs and have no spring in their steps, movement in their calves

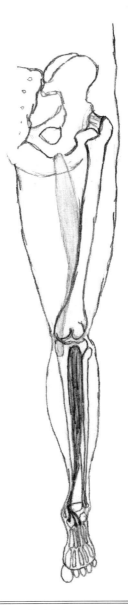

Figure 1.4 Tibialis posterior ascending to inner hamstring

or energy in their bodies—no movement in their toe hinges. Tiptoers seem to barely touch the ground when they walk…they really do look like they're trying to get across the room, the parking lot, or space, as fast as possible without touching the earth. Their energy is pent-up and their toe hinges won't let the entire foot touch the ground. It's a rare person who has the walk I think we all want to develop; the entire foot reaches the ground, then toes lift and spring us into the next step. Ankles are soft, and weight goes through and lifts from a spot behind the big toe. The foot experiences and enjoys the earth. Every step is a massage of the entire body above; energy flows.

A NEW WALK

So let's walk. Experiment with walking slowly with less weight in your heels, and *springing* from that spot behind the big toe with every step. I've found that as I push myself up and off from my big toe and inner arch *slowly*, I wake up my core line.

I walk with the head up and keep my low back open—back and relaxed. I let my knees flex and stay open, and I ask the toe hinges to stay flexible and springy *while* I allow myself to sink into my legs and feet with each step. I truly want my foot to touch the ground. If part of my foot hesitates to contact the ground, I make a conscious effort to live in that spot a bit more fully. I ask the toe hinge to open and *stay* resilient. As I work the toe hinge, I feel its pumping action adding energy all through my body.

Allow yourself to observe the feelings of movement or stagnation when you walk, and exaggerate both settling

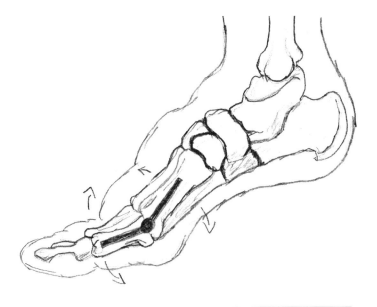

Figure 1.5 *Too many of us aren't aware we're supposed to have a big toe hinge*

into *and* springing through the feet, legs, and knees. Notice if you shorten and tighten your back, land heavily in your heels, or forget to spring off. Put more energy into lifting your body with your toes to massage your entire deep line of muscles. Realize that walking awareness is something you can practice anywhere and everywhere without it being too obvious that you're working to reclaim your body.

In 2006 I caught a loose shoelace at the top of an escalator and pitched forward very hard, landing on my right knee. I dislocated the smaller outside bone of the leg; I bruised my kneecap and jarred my body all the way up into my hip and back. I couldn't bend my knee or even bring it close to my body. For six months, I lost the ability to lift myself onto my toes unless I grabbed onto a support and pulled myself up with upper body strength.

I worked with many practitioners—and I know lots!—on both sides of the Atlantic. No one could help me rehabilitate that knee. I decided to practice what I preach. In addition to my regular rebounder program, I started doing what I call "big toe pushups". I simply stood still; then I worked to lift myself up using big toes only.

BIG TOE PUSHUPS

If you try this pushup concept for yourself, chances are you'll notice that when you lift into your toes, your foot turns out a bit (see Figure 1.6) and the weight transfers into your little toes as you lift. Your toe hinges are no longer horizontal. Lifting with the smaller toes makes the hinge open and point toward the outside. But we want to strive for horizontality of the hinge. This sideways pushup creates a high inner arch in both feet, or perhaps one foot more than the other. It causes us to lose that horizontal hinge.

I didn't want this to happen—I wanted to feel the lift in the big toe (see Figure 1.7). Sure enough, when I focused on lifting and controlling the hinge from the big toe, I felt energy (and discomfort!) in my knee, hip, and back. *Suddenly by working my toe hinge, I could feel hinges all the way up my body!* I felt a deep-seated tension and weakness, a lack of life, through the core of my being. I could feel that deep leg muscle complain with every lift. I began working the damaged leg by holding my other leg completely off the ground and asking the big toe of the damaged

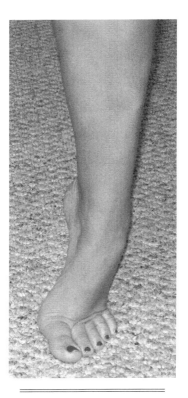

Figure 1.6 The toe hinge
pushing to the outside

right leg to lift me. At first I *had* to hold onto something to allow my arms to lift me up through those non-firing muscles.

I did a few of these big toe lifts whenever I had a chance—at the post office, on the phone, in the morning. Eventually I put less of the work in my arms and more of the lift right down in my big toe. Finally, one day I was able to stand on my right foot, lift my left foot off the ground, and raise myself up in my right big toe! The pain in my knee and my hip is now 95 percent gone.

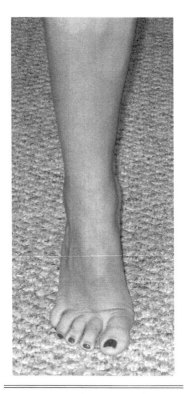

Figure 1.7 A horizontal big toe
hinge is most efficient

Toe pushups are as easy or difficult as you want to make
them. When you hold one foot completely off the ground
to lift with the other big toe, it's difficult. This workout needs no equipment. If your foot won't lift you yet,
just grab whatever support is available. When you have a
moment, come up into one big toe, then the other, then
both. Where you find the weakness, work it. How often
should you do this? Whenever you have a chance, try three
to ten of these lifts. I wouldn't do 50 or 100 at a time.
We're not after bulk, we're after awareness. It's absolutely

worked for me, and given me back my legs. Currently, this is a favorite exercise!

USING STEPS

Climbing steps in toe pushup fashion has shown me how hard I work to protect my knees. We'll cover the knee hinge in a later chapter, but consider that perhaps most of us don't have bad knees—we have bad hips, ankles, legs, and toes that try to protect knees, with the result that the knees stop functioning properly.

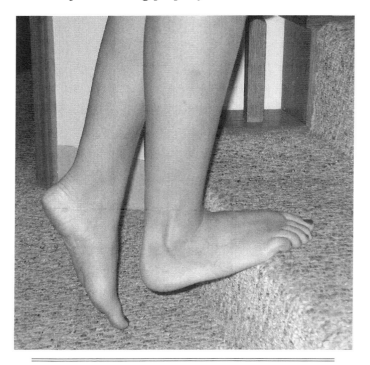

Figure 1.8 Sinking into stairs allows the deep line to waken

When I remember to climb in slow motion and stay aware of every subtle movement beginning in my toes, my knees hurt, but feel awakened. Once you *decide to lift yourself up and down the stairs with the core instead of hauling yourself by the external muscles*, you really begin to find your deep line. I allow my heel to sink down past the stair tread, then work to lift myself onto the riser, using the toe hinge and the core of my leg. Even if you can't lift yourself and find you're only able to sink into the step, if you decide to stretch your foot as you relax into the step, you're at least beginning to challenge the leg muscles. You're waking up your legs. Pay attention to the tracks of your knees; keep them as straight ahead as possible. Make steps be a light workout for you, and *enjoy them*!

I absolutely believe that if we'd learn to slow down, feel more of our bodies and their movements, and allow ourselves to experiment with identifying and learning to use all our muscles, we'd live in a far different world. Start with your toes and work your way up the body. Using any of the ideas we've discussed, slowly and mindfully, gives you an entirely new workout. And if you can remember to do it joyfully, your bodymindcore will appreciate the shift.

So in a perfect world, we'd neither be "set back on our heels" or "tiptoeing through minefields". We'd be able to walk, securely, yet with a spring in our step. We'd find that spot behind the big toe, sink into and spring from it. Each step would invite our big toe hinge to oil itself, to work itself, and to spring our entire body through life. What are we waiting for?

⊣ THE ANKLE HINGE ⊢

A FIRM FOUNDATION?

So much of what goes wrong in our world and our bodies could be corrected if we only had a firm foundation! When our ankles won't find a horizontal position, we can't plant our feet firmly on the ground. We "dig in our heels" to survive whatever we expect the world will give us. When that happens, we're not "standing our ground", and we can't be happy in our lives. Let's see what we can do to change this.

It's been twenty years since I survived the plane wreck that put me in the back pain club. Because of my fused spine, I work harder than most people to keep reasonably pain free. The gift of knowing back pain intimately has allowed me to understand pain in a way that's changed me and many others as well. I'm starting to comprehend bodymindcore deeply, and my bodywork students have noticed lately that my fused spine is beginning to show quite a curve. That's an exciting validation of my work and my thinking.

Remember how I divide us all into three groups: those who pull their energy up into their cores because of fear of the unknown, those who've collapsed at the core and allow their energy to sink into the earth because of defeat, and those few who are energized at the core and have a joyous "spring in their step"? I'd like to help everyone see how they might join this latter group, and one of the main changes will come from the ankle hinge.

A HORIZONTAL HINGE

In this chapter we'll look more closely at a horizontal ankle hinge. As you look at the ankle from the back, you begin to understand our problem. The flat footed, the plodders (Figure 2.1), often have an inner ankle bone that's level to or just a bit higher than the outer bone. Their inner ankle "bump" will peer toward the inside floor. Actually the outer bone should be fairly level with the inner; in a flat foot it's often not. A person who lurches through the world on high arches—perhaps someone who had dance training early on (Figure 2.2)—will have a hinge where this inside ankle bone is actually quite a bit higher than the outer, instead of slightly higher.

In an efficient ankle hinge, the inner bone will probably be slightly higher, but will approach a horizontal hinge. What we want to create is the most efficient, most level, most useable ankle hinge we can find. This way we're not collapsing inner or outer arch; we're not crumbling our foundation in a way that causes all the blocks above to no longer fit together efficiently.

I chose to talk about toe hinges as if there was only one plane of movement—up and down, through the big toe. Clearly this isn't totally accurate: When we lift into

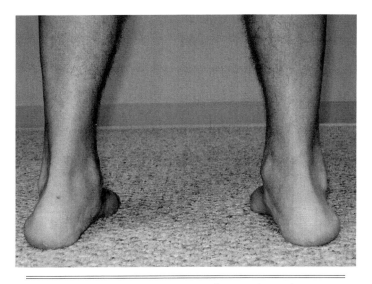

Figure 2.1 A collapsed inner arch; weight in the center line

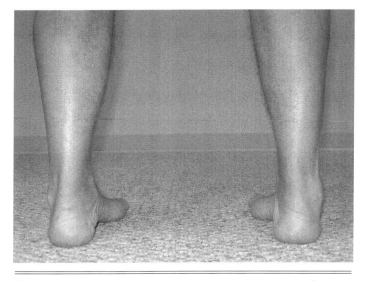

Figure 2.2 An inner arch too high at the center; collapsed on the outer arch

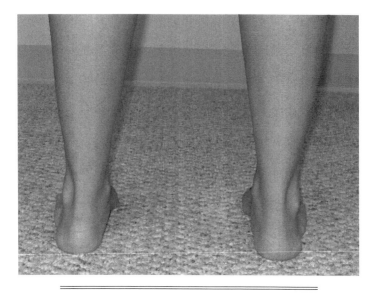

Figure 2.3 Balanced arches, balanced body

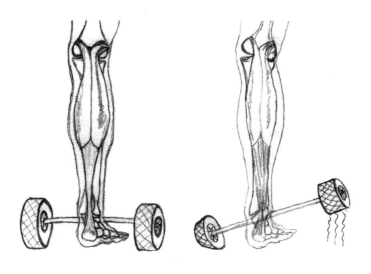

Figure 2.4 Ankle bones and ankle hinges want to be level

our smaller toes instead of the big toe, we've changed the direction or horizontality of the hinge. The ankle hinge can have different personalities. See the two ankle bones as two wheels connected by an axle. Realize some of us are driving with one wheel down on the shoulder or up on a curb (Figure 2.4).

The hinge sits on an axle that can move side to side as wheels move independently of each other. It's hard to find the horizontal hinge we're after until we get these ankle bones to horizontalize.

As we work up through the body we'll find many hinges that operate in more than one direction. But ankle hinges, like any others, will operate better the more they're aligned and oiled. If we're operating a hinge that's not on the horizontal plane, and if we're walking and standing with most of our weight in our heels instead of toes, we're going to have a tight, tired, inefficient hinge. This tension may translate further up the body into knee problems, hip or low back problems; even neck and shoulder issues. We get well as we change this pattern and retrain our ankles.

Taken together, the toe and ankle hinges are in charge of health all the way through the body. The legs are full of veins that return blood back up to the heart. They have no mechanism to send blood back to the heart, *except the pumping action of the calf muscles*. When we plod on stale feet and legs, no deep muscle moves the blood back up through the trap doors of the veins. If we're heavy in our heels, we're not pumping any of the old blood away. But every time we step into and through our ankles and toes with purpose, we've just milked that old blood further up our legs toward our lungs and heart, as well as getting our lymphatic system to flush. Let's learn to stretch the calves.

WHAT'S THE BEST WAY TO STRETCH?

How do we stretch effectively? Some experts tell us to never hold a stretch for more than three to five seconds. Others tell us to always hold at least twenty seconds. Who's right? Both are. Each teacher has a specific reason for what he or she teaches, and their reasons all make sense. Here's my method and here are my reasons.

I don't set a time frame on how long one should hold a stretch. I suggest you find a stretch, breathe into it, and continue to work with it *as long as you feel you're unwinding comfortably*. Hold until you easily feel breath move through the place you're stretching. Then release. If you work too long or hard, you'll anger tissue; but if you truly listen to your body, you'll continue to unwind pieces of the deep line at an appropriate rate. This nebulous instruction frustrates some clients, but I don't want to become anyone's doctor or guru; I want us all to realize we're our own best authority. Personally, I often take a stretch into a "cramp" and work to relax into and release that cramp. This works for me. Common sense is the benchmark here, always.

Often I give clients the image of a rubber band. When you hold only one end of the band, it's hard to stretch it. Hold both ends. What if you also twisted the ends of the band as you stretched it long, and even found a way to stretch the middle of the band in yet another direction? Can you see how each different direction of stretch contributes to the ability of the whole rubber band to lengthen and become resilient?

IT'S CALLED "CONNECTIVE" TISSUE

Our muscles and their wrappings, our fascia or connective tissue network, are like a rubber band. The more directions we create when we stretch, the more we wake the entire body. I'll often ask a client on my treatment table to lengthen an inner leg and heel, *while* pulling the low back into the table, *while* bringing the chin toward the chest, *while* remembering to breathe! The more I get the client to work, the more he or she releases. The same will be true for you as you work with these stretches. Find more directions to ask your body to stretch, all at the same time, and breathe!

When one begins to look for lines of transmission, one realizes that every part of the body is connected by muscle and fascia or connective tissue to every other part. This tissue wraps muscle groups, individual muscles, and even sections of muscles. All our hinges through the body are on the same road. Stretching any one area will change the entire body—above or below. The tibialis posterior, that deep leg muscle right behind the bones, will lose its resiliency if it's not asked to work. If we don't have spring in our step, the muscle acts as deep, dried glue or hard taffy that knits the bones together. Whether we plod *or* pull our arches high, the calf isn't exercised with each step the way it's designed to be worked. And when there's no resiliency in the deep leg, knees are stiff and painful too. Clear the feet and legs; open everything above.

SIMPLE KNEE BENDS

How do we create, or approximate, this horizontal ankle hinge? The first and easiest way is by a simple knee bend. Place both feet pointing straight ahead, about sitting-bone width apart—perhaps six to eight inches. Now, begin mild knee bends. You're going to try to watch several things at once: Are your feet remaining fairly straight, or does one sneak off to a side? Does one or do both inner arches creep up off the floor as you bend your knees? What about your heels? Do your knees track straight ahead, or do they likewise get off track? And last, how horizontal does your ankle hinge remain as you do this work? Are you driving with one wheel in the gutter? Remember how in the previous chapter we checked into the six separate points on the foot, to see if we were balancing among them? This is again the first important step to finding a clean ankle hinge. Redistribute the weight of your foot among all six points as you practice knee bends.

I've been experimenting with these knee bends for quite some time and find I really have learned to put energy in my whole body by simply raising and lowering my upper body through the knees while remembering to keep my ankles horizontal and my low back relaxed. I invite you to feel the different points in your foot—big toe, small toe, inner heel, outer heel, inner arch, outer arch—and experiment with allowing weight to anchor in each of these spots individually as you knee bend. I think you'll feel a shift above, in the muscles of your legs, as you experiment with different weight bearing. Chances are you'll also find spots where you don't like to rest your weight. These are the spots I suggest you give the most attention, because they're telling you where you haven't been living. We'll talk more about the knees in the next chapter; for now work your knees to work your ankle hinges.

Are you ready to add another challenge? What happens in your body if you practice these knee bends to keep the ankle hinge free and horizontal, *while you're gently exercising and using your toe hinge at the same time?* Allow yourself to slightly lift into your toes at the same time you bend your knees just a bit. Can you feel how, again, you're waking up muscles higher in the body? Can you begin to see how happy feet will give us happy bodies above?

Remember our mindful walking in the last chapter? We're going to give our gait a new focus: a horizontal ankle hinge added to the use of a horizontal big toe hinge, which keeps us from striking too heavily in our heels. *As we learn to lift our bodies with our toe hinges while we keep the ankle both resilient (not striking the ground heavily) and level, we'll find a new body above.*

BAREFOOT WALKING

I've begun to enjoy barefoot walking. I lower my center of gravity so that with each step my knees are bent and I'm slightly crouched. I don't worry about whether heels touch first, the foot rolls heel to toe, or any of those cues I've heard. I just ask the entire foot to reach for the ground and spread when it touches, flattens into and pushes off the ground. I visualize my four points of the foot sinking into and staying longer on the ground with each step; then I find that magic spot behind the big toe and work to *spring* from it and push off with every step.

Occasionally I'll slow down my weight transfer enough to find an old or weak spot I hadn't realized was still bothering me. During this step I also pay attention to the ankle—do I overuse or underuse my toe hinges? Or do I spring through the toes with the heel happily following along? I do this *very* slowly. It's amazing how your walk and your body change if you'll stay with this pattern awhile.

I'm not a fan of orthotics or any sort of appliance that holds the foot where it should be. To me they're a crutch. While I may use crutches on a short term basis, I'd like to learn how to throw them away. If nothing but orthotics will serve you, use them; but remember, they're still crutches. How can you learn to strengthen your feet and legs to let your crutches go?

EARLY WALKERS

Years ago I watched a client walk after a particularly deep session, and asked, "Did you walk early when you were a baby?" As she crossed the room she lurched…she toddled. She told me she'd walked at nine months; the next day she called to tell me her older sister said it was actually six months when she'd begun walking. Think about this: When we stand and learn to hurtle ourselves across the room to our goal, it works. We're up and moving forward. Why change what works? Yet at some point, wouldn't it be good to realize that we lurch across the room and to learn to slow down, let our feet touch the ground, and retrain our body to enjoy walking as we find efficiency?

After my wreck I probably walked too soon. It was

important to me to know I could get back on my feet. One practitioner friend recently said, "You are wired *so* strangely!" I know what she means. I've spent twenty years powering through life without paying attention to the damaged areas. Now as I slow down to feel the damaged deep line and invite awareness to return, resiliency and life are coming back to my body. Meeting your body can be painful, but it's exciting! Occasionally a muscle complains or even goes on strike, but I can tell I'm letting go of fear and self-punishments and living more happily in my feet and my body.

How else can we "oil" our ankle hinges? In addition to the above knee bends, here are several simple things you can do to ask the ankles to wake up. Sit or lie on the floor or a chair or bed, point your toes; then draw circles with the toes while stretching ankle hinges, or even writing your name with your toes. Remember you're trying to really stretch your ankles, so perhaps you want to write your name with your toe pointing back toward your forehead! I'm constantly experimenting with new positions. I'll lie in bed on my side, pull my big toe as far away from my body as possible, then stretch and draw circles. With this stretch I'm already working with hinges farther up the line. See if you can feel the deep muscle in the calf release. I'll literally stretch until I feel cramping; I work right into the cramp, hold on and breathe as I try to release the pain. I can't over-emphasize how effective simple stretching can be.

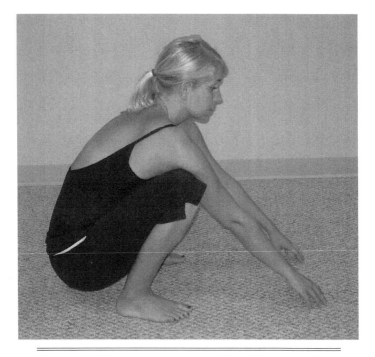

Figure 2.5 Practice squatting while shifting weight to
various points of the feet

SQUATS

Here's another way to change feet and legs: *squat* while
keeping feet flat into the floor as you go down. Can you
feel how leaving your heels on the ground stretches both
your legs and these ankle hinges? Can you feel how your
big toe is challenged to stay balanced and remain on the
floor? For many of us, it's hard to maintain this position,
yet many cultures live much of their lives in this squat and
have far fewer problems with backs, bellies and bodies in
general than we do.

Learning to squat while keeping the feet flat, *and shifting your weight from foot to foot,* will change everything above. Remember to keep your feet pointed straight ahead! Realize you're stretching a line which begins at the under surface of the foot and travels all the way to the back of your head. Stay in this position and experiment with finding new spaces.

As we work through the body, I'm going to encourage you with each chapter, to relate what we're doing in any hinge to all the hinges above and below. Though we're dividing the body into segments, remember we're finding one continuous core line, no matter where we do our work. I'd like to convince you that shifting anything will shift everything; then get you to shift toward a healthier and happier body.

This chapter asks you to think about how you relate to the earth and move through a secure universe. Too many of us aren't satisfied on the planet in this time; we don't let our feet, or our core, touch the ground. We're either wound too tightly or we're defeated. By asking you to consider a middle ground which changes the way your toes and heels relate to the earth, *I'm challenging you to change the way you relate to yourself and others as you move through the world.* You can hold your breath, suck up your energy and tiptoe through life; you can plod through a joyless life; or you can put a spring in your step and see each foot you place on the path as a joyous moving forward in the universe. The choice is yours.

⊣ THE KNEE HINGE ⊢

INFLEXIBILITY AND FEAR

Too many of us have troubles with our knees. Often, every other part of the body works great, but our knees just don't seem to want to support us. I've found over the past quarter century's work that while I don't feel I do miracle work on the knees, I do acceptable work on the feet, ankles, and hips; the knees often get better. This statement returns to a concept which you may get tired of hearing about: tracking. It's the goal of this chapter to create free knee hinges that operate on a clear track. We're going to see the knees as one of the rustier and least-used hinges of the body, and see if we can oil them to create true resiliency and efficient movement.

Louise Hay wrote *You Can Heal Your Life* (1984, Santa Monica, CA: Hay House Publishing), which I find to contain some intriguing ideas. Basically she correlates body parts and disease conditions to emotional maladies. For example, she claims that arthritis is often caused by underlying resentments stored in the body. She suggests nearly every condition can be traced to its deepest level: "I'm not

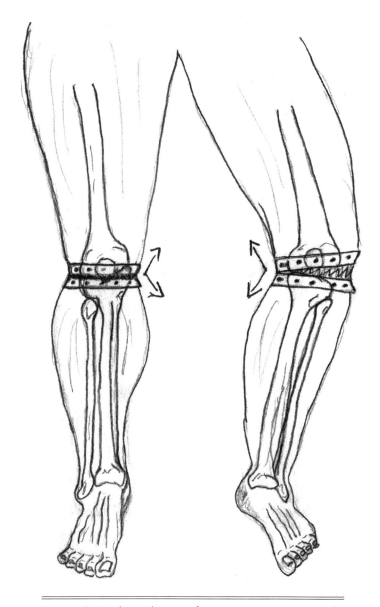

Figure 3.1 A knee hinge often operates in a straight forward/back line. Right: It can also swivel or twist slightly off this line

good enough." I think she's on to something, even if I don't agree with all her conclusions.

Her statement about knees is interesting. She suggests they represent inflexibility, inability to give in or to bend: fear. If you're having problems with your knees, this may be something for you to consider. *How could I move through life more joyfully, allowing life to flow through me and my knees? How could I learn to be a more flexible person?*

In previous chapters we mentioned some of the old sayings we've all heard or used. We hear of someone or something that makes us "weak in the knees". We seem to confuse "weakness" in the knees with knee flexibility and resiliency, however. I have doubts about the benefits of being "strong in the knees", because I feel strength doesn't denote flexibility. I'd like us all to realize the knee hinge and its effective use could change all hinges above and below, again, simply by developing tone in this area.

Too many clients of my age and even younger are experiencing replacement surgeries of their knee joint. Why? It's because we don't know how to use, stretch, and oil our knee hinges. The more we learn to unwind our deep lines, toes to head, the more we'll soften the knees, remove the pain and stiffness. Let's look further.

LOCK YOUR KNEES

Often I'll stand a new client in my treatment room so I can observe his or her stance. Many times, if I suggest to a client "lock your knees", we both realize the knees are already locked! There's no energy in the joint at all. How

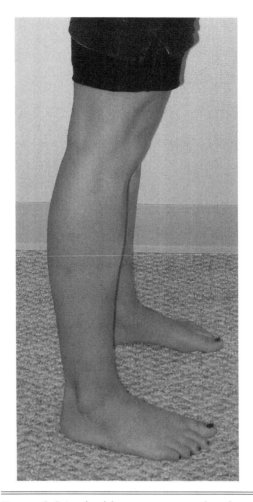

*Figure 3.2 Locked knees cause a slowdown
of energy through the entire body*

can energy move through a line where the tissue's totally
tensed?

I encourage the client to slightly flex or bend the
knees. Many clients feel unsteady as they allow the knees
to soften; after reflection, they often realize their low backs

feel easier and their feet touch the ground differently. Let me point out again how a locked knee also makes it far more difficult for blood and old toxic wastes to travel up from the feet on their way to the liver for cleansing and replenishing. Unlock your knees, be flexible and add another shock absorbing hinge to your body.

Sometimes I'll also encourage a client to lock their knees while they're performing a stretch. My reasoning is this: With locked knee joints/hinges, the client is able to stretch and extend the entire line from feet to head. When they soften the knee joint, it takes stress away from the stretch. I believe a bit of stress is good, and by tightening and softening each hinge, including the knees, clients begin to relax their tension and their fears. They're discarding pain and inflexibility.

WHY DO WE HAVE PAIN?

Pain is such an interesting topic. Many of us live in pain: mental, physical, or emotional pain which robs us of our energy to perform daily activities. If it hurts to get out of bed, we're prone to lie in bed longer. If it hurts to sit at the computer, we're likely to put off work that has to be done. If we're in a hurtful relationship, we hold our breath, tiptoe through, and hope for the best. *We'll deny our pain its opportunity to tell us to make changes and, at the end of the day, we hurt even more.* We try to modify, mollify or stifle too much of our pain instead of listening to it to understand how we might clean it out of our bodies.

HOW MUCH LOVE?

Years ago I attended a seminar and private session with Rev. Bryan Graham, a Unity minister who at that time lived in Florida and traveled around the country presenting workshops. His critical question to participants was, *"How much love are you willing to allow in your life?"* I've often wondered whether he knows how his work changed lives. This question relates for me to another: How hard must you work to keep your knees locked? Do you see a relationship?

Ask yourself: Who do you still try to please (but rarely succeed) by whatever self-punishing behaviors you've chosen? Who still controls you? One or both parents? Grandparents or siblings? A primary caregiver or friend outside the family? A teacher? A boss? Are you trying to achieve standards you imagine these people had or still have for you that you will almost certainly fail to uphold? Putting some real thought into these questions can be profitable, especially if you persevere: What part of that futile behavior am I still choosing? Is it life enhancing? From here the questions come even faster: Am I genuinely honoring my role models with this behavior? Am I honoring me? Does it serve them, or me? Often the answer to all these last questions is "no". When you can answer these questions truthfully, you're on your way to unlocking your knees.

Now that we've stretched the mind, let's stretch the body. Here's an interesting test. Lie on your back. Bring both your knees in toward your body. Now, begin a bicycling motion, bringing first one knee, then the other toward your chest. Observe the tracking of your knees and feet. Does one knee or do both turn toward the outside? Do the feet turn inside or outside as knees approach the chest? Ask the knees and feet to draw straight lines as they come toward the chest. Do you feel tugs or pulls on muscles in other places? Ida Rolf gave us a simple idea that applies here: "Put it where you want it and ask it to move." You want your foot, ankle, knee and hip to all operate efficiently up and down the same line or track. Simply put things in the right place and practice moving with them in that efficient place.

ON TRACK, BACK TO THE STAIRS

I've found an effective way to wake up my knees is on stairs. I simply place one foot on the step, *allow my heel to sink down* below the stair, *and pull myself up* through that foot while I add mild stress in my knees as I work through the lift (Figure 3.3). I don't allow my "sleeve" muscles to pull me up, but focus on asking the deeper core muscles to raise me. I don't lock my knees or ask them to stay inflexible; I do ask them to work through a full range of motion. *And, I stay on top of myself—I don't bend forward as I'm climbing.*

Often I don't even climb the stairs; I just bounce up and down with toes, ankles, and knees. I happily use the railings; I even allow myself to do some of the work of climbing through my arms in addition to my legs, when necessary. But I work to engage my deep line with every step. I find if I climb several flights of steps a day with this mindful attitude, my knees feel oiled.

Coming down steps, I again encourage my knee to get involved in the process. When a foot lands on a stair, I then ask my weight to transfer to this stair through my knee. If

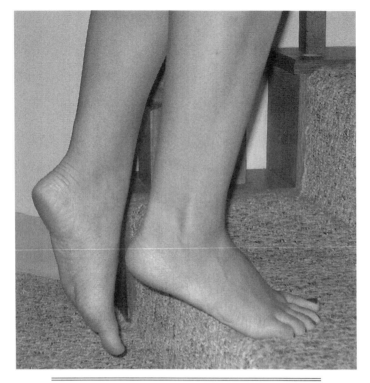

Figure 3.3 Allow the heel to sink, then pull the
weight up through the knee and entire leg

each step up or down asks the knees to "use it or lose it",
chances are we'll learn to use them more fully and prolong
their lives. You may realize, as I have, that when we keep
the weight-bearing focus in our knee, all the way down to
the step, we wake a hinge that hasn't known how to allow
weight to move through it. This is an important idea: we
truly have lost our knees through dis-use.

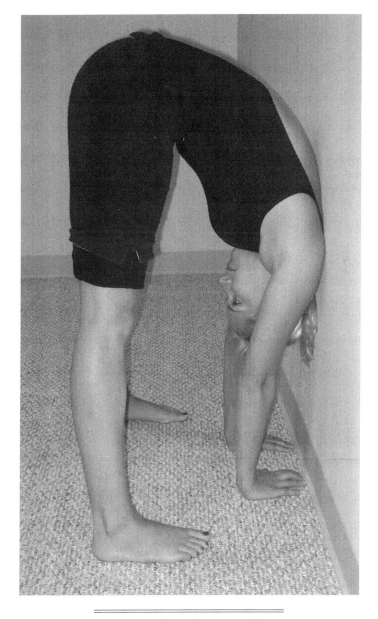

Figure 3.4 The "downward dog"
yoga posture, against a wall

MY FAVORITE EXERCISE

My favorite exercise to encourage my deep holding patterns to unwind is what I call a "downward dog with resistance". *If I only have time for one minute of stretching per day, I use this yoga posture to ask my entire body to stay open.* I feel I can stretch all my hinges at once, and I'm absolutely oiling my knee hinges. I specifically ask the inner hamstring on the leg to stretch out of both the calf and the back in the traditional downward dog posture. I modify this posture by lowering my head as I slide it down *against a wall* (Figure 3.4). Perhaps you'll find this posture is too difficult for your body. Here's a suggestion: Face an armchair, put your hands on the arms, and try the stretch with the support of the chair. Even clients with very fragile backs can often achieve a bit of stretch and rehabilitation with this modified posture.

I stand with my toes perhaps twelve to sixteen inches from the wall, then bend forward and let the back of my head travel down the wall toward the floor. I'm not trying to touch the floor with my head. I'm trying to feel a stretch in the neck, the middle and low back, and calf; but most specifically in the *inner hamstring,* just above my locked knees. This deep muscle often gets overlooked when we stretch.

In the last year inner hamstrings have climbed my list of the spots where I believe we can make the most change in a body by putting energy into a specific site. I believe it's the first muscle to challenge when we're ready to change the "stand your ground" and "lock your knees" mentality.

As you move into this forward position to isolate your inner hamstring, point your feet inward to stand pigeon-

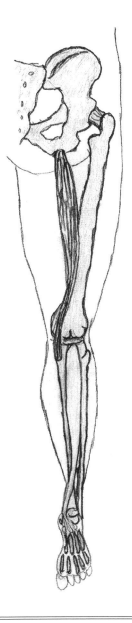

Figure 3.5 The inner hamstring connects the knee to the hip

toed. As you now bend, do you feel additional stretch in your inner hamstrings and additional stress in your knees? Push the inner arches of your feet into the floor. If you pay attention as you bend further forward you'll feel the arches try to pull up into your legs. By staying grounded you're stretching the toe hinge out of the lumbosacral hinge which we'll discuss soon. And as you do, you're stretching and oiling the knee hinge. You'll doubtless feel a stretch on the back and inside of the legs; you may feel a burn from short, tight connective tissue that's finally starting to loosen. Remember, a little burn is a good thing—a lot is too much, possibly even tearing tissue instead of releasing it. You didn't get this tied up in ten minutes; why should everything let go in that time?

Here's a stretch to open not only the knee hinge, but every hinge up and down the back. It's another hamstring stretch. We're stretching from the sitting bones at the back of the thigh, and down to the back and side of the knees. Lie on your back. Use a belt, rope, or stretching cord. Place it across the middle arch of your foot. Now, straighten your leg and pull this entire straightened leg, thigh and knee line toward both the ceiling and your body. Keep your hip anchored into the floor or bed. As you do, you'll feel some stretch at the back of your knee, but also up the hamstrings, into the low and middle back, and at the ankle. If you even bring the toes toward the floor, you'll find you're stretching muscles all the way up and down your hinges. Again, use common sense. You're not trying to tear tissue; you're trying to stretch it.

Lie back on the floor with both feet in front of you. Then drag one foot around behind you so it's near your hip. Continue to sit back, rock back, and encourage the knee to begin pulling out of the lower leg, but also the hips and the spine. Remember, it's important to expand the breath. We'll talk more about breathing in Chapter 7.

ON THE REBOUNDER

My preferred fitness program works my entire deep line by focusing on the knees, calves and feet. I have a rebounder, a small trampoline three feet in diameter and six inches off the ground. I work with this equipment for about twenty minutes most mornings.

I never bounce totally off the surface; my toes always stay on the material. I work the backs of my calves, create flexibility in my toe hinges, exercise my knees, and

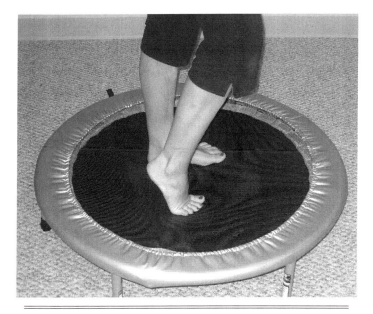

Figure 3.6 Using a rebounder for ankle hinge resiliency

increase the circulation all through my body. When I miss several days I feel the difference. You can usually find this rebounder in the sporting goods section of department stores. It's the most cost-effective piece of exercise equipment I've found. If you really want a workout, add the earlier toe pushups. About ten toe lifts may wear you out!

NOW, GET CREATIVE WITH THIS HINGE

Again, find the six spots on the base of your foot from Chapter 1 and divide your weight equally among them. Put most of your weight in the big toe; then do a slight knee bend and feel the muscles up your calf. Move to the inner arch spot, and knee bend again. Work all six spots, and when you find a connection that's weak, work that spot a bit more. This is as easy or difficult as you want it to be. It's a slightly different exercise in this chapter because you're now focused on what's happening, or not happening, at the knees. And remember how feeling toe and ankle hinges at the same time really begins to unwind the entire line from feet to head.

Let's add another concept: Can you do a knee bend on one leg only, asking your other foot to remain off the ground? Lift one foot, but ask the second foot to carry you into and through the knee bend. What's happening? Do you feel weakness through the leg? Can you ask that weakness to support you more fully? What happens as you even lift yourself into the toes, working your toe hinge, ankle hinge, and knee hinge all at the same time? Let's oil the entire line! Remember, it's all right to hold onto a counter or railing as you learn to awaken this line.

KNEE CIRCLES

I've found lately I'm really enjoying drawing circles or figure "U"s reaching forward, with both knees *at the same time*, and in a mild knee bend fashion. Stand with feet straight on and sitting-bone width apart. Allow both knees to begin describing circles or "U"s—forward, outside, back, inside. What you're trying to feel is movement in both your feet and knees. Remember to take the circle in the opposite direction too. And again, when you feel yourself favoring a spot, stop to explore! One reason I like this work: I realize I'm stretching the knee hinge away from and out of the ankle hinge. Can you feel it? You'll feel how the knee hinge isn't always a simple forward-and-back hinge either. All our hinges are more complicated than that.

Can you see how most of the exercises from previous chapters work the knee hinge? Squats, knee bends, stairs and toe pushups all give the knee hinge a good workout. We've just turned the tables: where we've been working our way *up* the line to stretch the next hinge above, we're now stretching the lower hinges out of higher ones as well. You'll find different tight spots depending on the direction of your intention. We often use the phrase "Use it or lose it." I think there's truth in this phrase. I invite you to slow your movements, feel the weakness or strength in muscles, and learn to reawaken your line and hinges.

If we see the knees as one of the rustier of our hinges, if we decide to wake them up, pay attention to them all the way to the bodymindcore, and if we learn to trust them, I believe we'll change our worlds entirely. We'll learn flexibility, we'll learn resilience, and we'll learn to move through life in our chosen direction—happily.

THE HIP HINGES

In my textbook I talk about the seven backs of the body: foot, pelvic bowl, pelvic floor, gut, heart, arm, and head backs. Much of what I've written in that book for serious bodywork students is still useful information for the reader of this book. For example, a place we don't think about much is the pelvic bowl and its hip hinge; it's a spot we often gloss over or pretend doesn't exist, until it gives us trouble and we consider a hip replacement.

OUR FIRST BALL AND SOCKET

I'm specifically thinking of the ball and socket hinge joint of the hip, where the hip bone ties into the socket with soft tissue. Here we have yet another type of hinge. Where the toe and knee hinges approach a straight back-and-forth with a small amount of wobble, and the ankle is something like an axle which may or may not be moving on a level surface, the hip joint allows the hinge to swivel in many directions. Your thigh can not only move forward and back in a straight plane; it can also turn inside and outside in nearly any direction you can create.

You can almost visualize the two hip joints as a two-legged stand (the bones) on which the pelvic bowl balances.

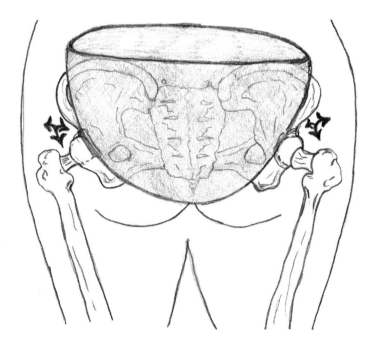

Figure 4.1 The hips and legs form a stand for the pelvic bowl

As we walk, first one leg stand, then the other, holds the stress of keeping the pelvic bowl in place. Many of us have too much tension in this hip hinge, causing a hip to tighten, to pull higher, or to be rotated forward or back. Most of us don't know our hips well; we need to get to know them better.

GIRD THE LOINS: IT'S THE ILIACUS!

Do you remember the Biblical term of "girding the loins"? I think that term denotes a tightening of this deep line— digging in the heels and pulling energy up to the pelvic bowl, all the way into the ribs and low back. If I just shorten my lower body up into this low back and "stand my ground", I'll survive. If I stay "on guard" against whatever dangers are coming my way, I survive. I gird my loins and face my foe. These phrases denote the idea that it's work to live in our feet. I'm suggesting as we follow this line above our feet we'll find that often *our feet don't touch the ground because we're holding our breath, girding our loins and standing our ground from far higher—the inside of the leg and hip.*

Why are our hips so tight? Louise Hay suggests that hip problems represent a fear of going forward in major decisions/directions. Perhaps there's some truth to this: like the priests in an earlier chapter, if we know where we want to go, won't we point our feet, ankles, knees, *and hips* in that direction? Yet, if we're fearful or uncertain about what we want, isn't it possible our tracks will likewise be scattered? And if we've been taught by elders not to feel our bodies or our needs, won't we find tension when we finally decide to pay attention to an area?

There's a deep muscle on the inside of the thigh that runs to the inside of the hipbone; in other words, a muscle from the leg to the hip that covers much of the hip hinge. It's called the *iliacus*, because it grows from the ilium or hip bone. When this muscle gets too tight, the leg, especially the inside, shortens into the hip and low back; the back tightens on that side.

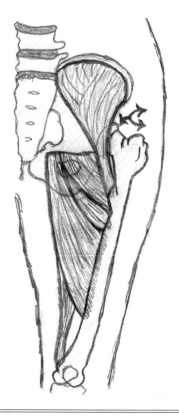

*Figure 4.2 The iliacus and adductor
muscles are key to healthy hips*

We need to learn to release this deep muscle that holds our
hips in place. A second muscle that holds the hip hinge
tight is down the inside of the leg. It's called the *adductor*.
As you can guess from its name, it *adds*, or brings together,
the legs. Can you see how tension in these two muscles
could contribute to hip pain, as well as pain further up
and down the body? Can you also consider that old sexual
traumas or other fears could tighten this area, causing pain
in muscles all the way to the bones?

LEVEL THE BOWL

I earlier mentioned the term "pelvic bowl". When the bowl isn't carried carefully and levelly, the contents spill out. This spillage is almost always toward the front of the body because we've tightened and lifted the sides and back of the bowl. The bowl is constructed with lots of bone on the back and the bottom, and very little at the front, so it's easy for the contents to spill forward when muscles weaken in the front and tighten in the back. That's what we'll try to correct with hip hinge stretches and later sacred hinge stretches. When we release this line inside the hip joint, we're on our way to revitalizing the pelvis and oiling the hip hinge.

FINDING THE DEEP LINE

How do we wake up this deep line of muscle? First and simplest, lie on your back, pull/push your low back into the floor or table, and try to extend/step down through your inner arch and heel. If you put a finger or thumb into the inside of your hipbone, you'll very possibly feel a tug, a tickle, or a sharp fear as you ask your inner arch to get longer. Suddenly you may have a direct experience of my contention that the feet touch the ground and settle onto the planet more happily when you remember to allow the hip hinge to release. Next, try marching in place: lengthen the opposite heel while pressing into the hipbone tissues; lengthen the same-side heel, back to the opposite, and so forth. As you work this line I think you'll find a new respect for the connection from foot to hipbone. I encourage you to explore this line for yourself, by yourself.

Remember knee bends from the previous chapter, where we focused on keeping knees moving forward in a straight plane? Let's experiment. As you bend this time, allow the feet to point to the outside instead of forward and allow your knees to follow the line of the foot and also point to the outside as you bend. Notice what's happening in your hips and tailbone. You may feel a tightening there. Now, put your feet and legs on straight and try the bend again. Can you feel your hips and sacrum soften and spread instead of tightening? Let's try even one more position—point your toes and knees in, then knee bend again. Do you feel a further opening/softening in your hip hinge area?

Z POSITION

A stretch I like to use to open the inside of the hip is what Rolfers call the Z position, based on a session from the advanced series of Rolfing work created by Emmett Hutchins and Peter Melchior. In this position, the client sits on the floor with both feet and knees in front of the body, pointing to the same side. In other words, the feet and legs make a Z.

He or she then pushes both knees toward the floor. When sitting in this position, the goal is to ask both sitting bones to touch the ground equally, while the spine grows straight and the back of the head also fits on straight (impossible). For most people the sitting bone on the side where the feet rest won't touch the ground

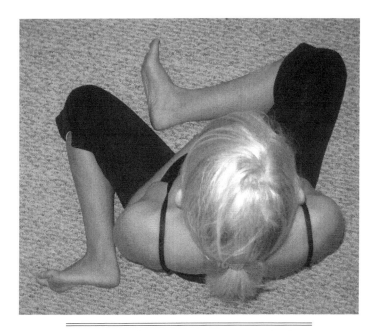

Figure 4.3 The Z position to open the hips

as easily. Sit in this position until tissues relax and settle toward the floor. As the high sitting bone sinks, the spinal line grows straighter, and the back of the head and neck also lengthen. The goal of creating as much length as possible really shifts the pelvic bowl back and asks the "immobile" sacroiliac joints to loosen. You've also begun to stretch your head hinge from your hip hinges, though we've not reached the top of the body yet! While you obviously would work harder on a tighter hip, remember to work both sides at all times.

To make a different stretch which may find yet another tension in your hip, next let your upper body simply lie back, or even draw circles with your upper body, while you continue to sit with your legs in the Z position. Remember, it's not as important to reach the floor with your shoulder as it is to feel a *mild* stretch all the way.

FINDING THE INSIDE OF YOUR LEGS

Now that we're in the pelvic floor and hip hinge, let's stretch the muscles inside the thigh out of the pelvis. Lie on your back with your tailbone up against the wall, and place your feet on the wall, toward the ceiling.

Allow your legs to spread out along the wall as your back stays on the floor and your sitting bones stay against

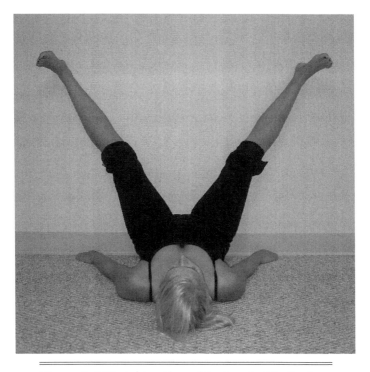

Figure 4.4 Stretching the adductors inside the legs

the wall. Stretch the legs out of the pelvis: open your low body up from the inside with this stretch. Breathe. Tighten and relax. Tighten and relax. Focus on the energy moving through your pelvis. Don't do anything with it; just observe. Stretch. Breathe. Relax. Feel.

Here's another, more forceful adductor stretch (Figure 4.5). Lie face down. Now come to a hands and knees position. Slide your knees along the floor, away from you, straight out to the sides as you sink your body into the floor. As much as possible, keep your knees as well as your hips (highly unlikely) and your ankles (fairly unlikely) on the floor.

Now, continue to spread your knees and slide your belly into the floor as the insides of your legs open wider and wider while your feet stay together. Go to the point where you feel a good stretch, but not to the point where damage occurs. You'll be able to discern this place and you mustn't go to it. *This stretch could tear a groin muscle if you push too hard.*

Again, breathe, relax, feel the pelvis open; instead of fear energy and tense energy, back off the stretch just a bit and feel the sex energy, joy energy, and free energy. Breathe, hold your stretch, and continue to focus on energy running through you. You can explore even more specifically by keeping one knee and leg long and straight while the other again explores outer reaches—to the side, long, twisting, pulling out of the groin, and then tightening as the other leg takes over. Can you feel it finding other areas of your body? This may bring up old feelings, fears or memories. You may find you need a friend, a counselor, or some other therapist to help you work through the feelings that sometimes surface.

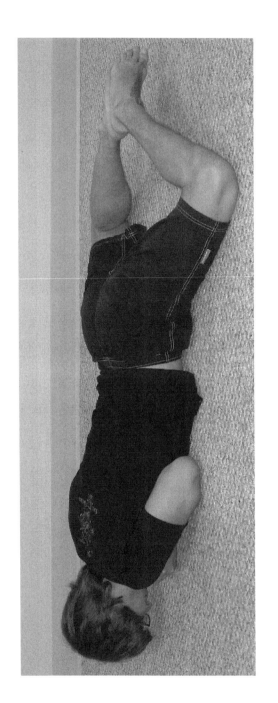

Figure 4.5 A more challenging stretch of the adductor compartment

TOO MUCH?

You can do a tamer version of the same stretch by lying on your back and allowing legs and knees to fall to the outside. Clearly, when you're face down, you're able to put more pressure onto the inner thigh compartment and the stretch is greater. But, just by lying on your back, relaxing the legs to the sides, and waiting for gravity to help you open the pelvis further, you'll begin to feel a softening. Remember, again: You don't need to go further and further. Simply stay with the stretch, the breath, and allow the legs to continue to find their way out and down.

But what if you really do have more congestion in one hip? In addition to the above "Z" position, here's an exercise I use. Try this: Lie flat on your back, dragging both knees slightly toward the ceiling, feet on the floor. Now, take your "good leg" and place the outside of the heel on the outside of the "bad hip" knee. Pull that knee across the center line of your body with your opposite foot while you push and hold your "bad" hip into the floor. In other words, you're going to use your foot to ask the knee hinge to pull to the inside in a way that stretches the outside and top of the hip hinge. Can you feel the stretch on the side of the leg and into the hip joint?

TICKLERS AND OTHER ABUSERS

Did you have a tickler when you grew up? Many of us had someone who enjoyed tickling us, and sometimes it was fun for both. However, too many ticklers are actually torturers. Many of us learned to tighten, shorten, and hold on until someone went away. Some of us are super-sensitive years later; others feel nothing because they're still holding their breath against their attacker. When tickling continues past the point where the receiver asks for the action to stop and isn't respected, it's no longer tickling; it's abuse. I was told by a counselor in a recent class that in some jurisdictions, tickling is now classified as abusive behavior.

Let's talk about sexual abuse. Years ago I attended a conference where a featured speaker suggested that three of every four women and one of two men had been sexually abused. I thought the figures were astoundingly high. They may or may not be accurate; I'm beginning to suspect they're more accurate than I first believed. Her point was that too many of us have suffered at the hands of an abuser.

What is an abuser? To me, it's someone who tries to gratify self at the expense of someone else and inappropriately uses power over them. With this definition, abuse leaves the sexual realm, and gives us all pause as to how and when *we've* become an abuser. But return to *sexual* abuse. When I realized that children are extremely *psychically* aware and have an intuitive sense that subconsciously knows when they're being misused, I understood that *nearly every child has been abused in the psychic realm.*

Many of us had someone older who gained their self-gratification at our expense, and when those psychic vibes came our way, we caught them even when we didn't understand them. We were left with feelings that something in our genital area was stirred; something about the stirring felt wrong. It wasn't *our* wrong! As children we couldn't know this, but many of us haven't been able to let go of these feelings of abuse. We're holding onto unresolved trauma in the hips and pelvic floor. It's time to release.

It's difficult for a young child who's been the recipient of sexual feelings from an older person to interpret the mixed messages their body gives. It's gratifying to be the object of an older person's attention! And often, a kind touch, or the thought of a kind touch in or around the genital area doesn't feel like a bad thing to a child. How confusing will a child's thoughts and feelings become when they're inappropriately touched, find a measure of pleasure in that touch; then feel a change in the energy and realize they're being hurt and mistreated by this elder from whom they still crave attention? Won't they tighten up in the hip joints?

FINDING THE PELVIC FLOOR

Some of us don't remember sexual abuses from childhood years. I'm not trying to create false memories for anyone, but I do strongly suggest that we've blocked much early sexual contact from our memories and consciousness, because *we didn't know what to do when sexualized touch came to us early and inappropriately.* We need to make it safe to go back into that past, deep into the bodymindcore and learn to *feel* the energy of the pelvis that too many of us learned to stifle long ago when someone looked or touched inappropriately. We often found that initial touch to be loving and reassuring; our world was upset when the touch became something else.

To find and tone our pelvic muscles and restore hip hinges, we borrow from Milton Kegel, a medical doctor who first used the following with patients. "Kegels" are simply stated: Tighten and relax the pelvic floor, to create tone. Repeat. Repeat. Another way to explain the exercise: Sit on the toilet and stop and start the flow of urine at least several times during urination, for different durations of time. Experiment with turning on and off the switch that controls your bladder release function; you'll also control the switch that turns on or off your sexual feeling/function. It's possible that switch has been stuck in "off" position for a long time. Many of us had situations around starting and stopping this flow in a performance situation (toilet training?) that may continue to affect the way we hold our pelvic floors, and our pelvic floor back, and our girded loins.

This exercise was found to be effective by Dr. Kegel in tightening and toning tissue, particularly in women. He used it primarily for two groups: women during and post pregnancy, and women with incontinence issues. He found positive changes in both groups. Today "Kegels" are often prescribed for both men and women to help them retrieve tone in the pelvic area. If done conscientiously, they're effective. Try "Kegels" whenever you have a chance—it can't hurt you.

NOW, CAN YOU RELAX?

Where I'd modify this exercise is by also focusing on the *relaxing* part of the work. Pay attention to the tightening, the strengthening, and the tension in the pelvic floor. At relaxation, *focus on the sensation of a free and sensual pelvis.* Now, switch back and forth—tense and relax/tense and relax. While maintaining these states for whatever time frame you choose, be it a few seconds to a couple of minutes in each phase, *learn to feel your feelings intensely "down there"* at the same time. Learn to find and feel your sexual energy, freely, with yourself before you share it with your partner. And since we all seem to need to judge ourselves, judge this energy to be good for you.

Ah, the pelvic floor. Whether from abuse of a sexual nature, a shaming experience around sex, a physical wreck or other trauma, beatings around the tailbone area, or plain fear of sexual energy and function, too many of us have lost the ability to lower our consciousness, our awareness, our *feeling nature* into the pelvis. We can't shake our hips. The hardest step for many when trying all the awareness exercises I'm recommending in this chapter is the step that says: *Feel your pelvis. Feel your sexual energy. Celebrate your sexual energy.*

Allow energy to move freely through your pelvis and throughout your body. To feel the pelvis goes against so many of the messages we received while we were growing up. We've been trained in a schizophrenic culture that suggests we need to be more sexual, yet also that we shouldn't be promiscuous. No wonder we all hold onto our pelvic floors! And by holding the pelvis, we're tightening the hip hinges. If one can let go, the other will follow. Loosen those hips.

CHAPTER 5

⊣ **THE SACRED HINGE** ⊢

STACKING BLOCKS ON A HOLY BONE

Do you remember stacking blocks as a child? Do you remember building a taller and taller stack, eventually to have the whole stack come tumbling down? Do you remember how, if you weren't careful, one low block out of line would cause a weakness and the whole stack fell? Or possibly the opposite happened: perhaps the last few blocks at the top got out of line and took the whole stack over with them as they tumbled.

Our spines are quite a bit like that stack of blocks; the more we keep them aligned, the more efficiently our spine stacks and the less likelihood of problems with or disintegration of the entire stack. And the foundation of this stack is the *lumbosacral junction.*

Although I'm calling it the sacred hinge, lumbosacrum is the place where the lumbar, or low back bones, join to the sacrum, or tailbone. This is one of the most important hinges in the entire spine. It's also a place few of us think about or give any attention at all, until it talks to us. Let's look more closely.

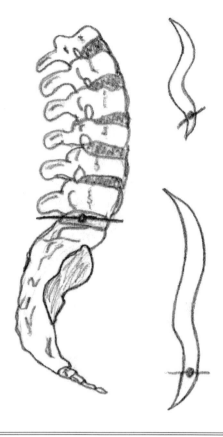

Figure 5.1 Lumbosacral hinge. The entire spine
is balanced on the sacrum and relationship
is critical. Upper right: a tipped lumbosacral
junction. Lower right: a level
lumbosacral junction

FINDING BALANCE

The sacrum was called the sacred bone in some cultures:
it's even been described as the seat of the soul. It's the

back of the pelvic bowl or basin described in the previous chapter, and the tail that flows from it. When this bone gets too tightly glued to the hipbones at the sacroiliac joints, there's no freedom in the pelvis. The more we keep movement in the sacrum and hips, the more we can keep the entire spine free and flowing. Visualize for yourself how the hip and lumbosacral hinges are two of all the hinges we have the most trouble learning to free.

DON'T WAG YOUR TAIL!

Think of a puppy dog that's just been disciplined for something its owner felt was wrong. What does a puppy almost always immediately do? It shortens its back and tucks its tail as far up between the legs and into the stomach as it can. You've watched this little play before. What happens within a minute? Have you seen a puppy in the middle of a scolding when its tail begins to slowly, surreptitiously waggle—incrementally at first, then soon in a fury of enthusiasm? Can you imagine how a puppy can be shamed at the front end and happy at the back at the same time? We need that talent. We need to learn that even if our head isn't on straight, we can feel relaxation and energy in our low back and pelvis. This awareness isn't even a stretch or exercise; it's a mental attitude. *Allow* the idea that your tail area could move freely. Don't work to make this happen; just allow.

I often tell clients as I work on their tailbone injuries (which nearly everyone has had) how I believe that the ligaments holding our tailbones in place are the vestigial remnants of tail-wagging muscles. I'm not trying to

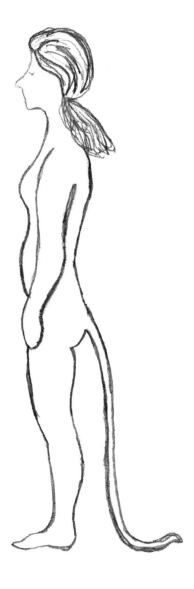

*Figure 5.2 Imagine you have a long, heavy tail
that reaches the ground and pulls your low back
down and back*

re-create muscles or offend anyone's beliefs, but I don't think we should mind if a tail decides to relax a bit and gently sway and be free. I even ask clients to stand and imagine they're the Pink Panther; imagine they have a long tail that drags the ground, where the tip finally chooses to wag. That's the feeling I'd like to elicit in terms of freeing the tailbone, for them, you, and me. This freedom even translates into more intense feelings in the genital area as we give ourselves permission to feel the feelings "down there".

Too many of us have had serious tailbone injuries, often forgotten. Some received brutal beatings or sexual abuse. Many have fallen down steps, or on skating rinks, or out of chairs. Nearly everyone I work with in a body-work setting can recall at least one or two tailbone traumas. Realize that these supposedly unrelated traumas can be part of the reason energy won't flow into your low back as freely as you'd like. Open, relax, breathe, and feel your tail. Let it loosen.

Picture the spinal bones. In all there are twenty-seven, *if* one counts the head bones as one, seven cervical or neck bones, twelve thoracic or chest bones, five lumbar or low back bones, one sacral or tailbone (that could actually be subdivided, and often is in younger people), and the tip of the tail, called the *coccyx*. These bones form the entire length of the spine, and are moved by their twenty-six hinges. Inside these spinal bones there's a channel the spinal column occupies, full of a tough tissue that coats the nervous network for the entire body. Whenever the bones get out of alignment, *something* slows. You can't allow two bones to fit together incorrectly without finding some kind of pinch or impingement on the nerves that travel the length of the spine and erupt at each hinge. When nerves get pinched, we suffer. Function is slowed, pain may result. It's our job to learn to stack our spinal blocks as efficiently as we can to prevent them from tumbling off and causing pain and loss of function.

Our sacred hinge is where the sacral bone or sacrum joins with and holds up the lowest lumbar vertebra or spinal bone. Like a juggler who balances a plate on a stick, this hinge, if in balance, really holds the entire spine happily. Too often, this hinge creeps forward, dumping the pelvis, and pinching the spinal column and nerves and causing pain in the low back. *If we can simply learn to keep our low back further back, we can often change the pain we're feeling in the back*; in addition we may even be able to bring feeling and function back into the hips and legs. If we can learn to hold the head and heart hinges open at the same time we're keeping the low back back, we've arrived. How do we do this? I just told you.

HEALTH IN THE DEEP FRONT MUSCLE

I believe we're sophisticated roly-poly bugs. Any trauma that comes at us, whether mental, emotional, physical, chemical, or energetic: all cause our body to shorten and tighten. There's a muscle on the front of the spine which travels to the inside of the leg; it's called psoas. For me, this muscle group is so involved in so many of the body's problems that I've named it Psoas, Storer Of All Stress.

It's the primary tightening mechanism for the front of the body; most of us, in response to fears, disappointments and challenges in our lives, shorten at least part of

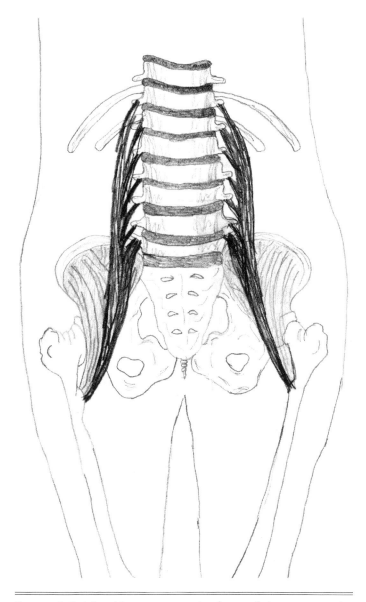

Figure 5.3 A healthy psoas on the front of the spine to the inside of the leg creates freedom in hip, sacred, stomach and heart hinges

the group in some way that in turn shortens or twists the fronts of our bodies, tightens and pulls forward one or both sides of our low backs, and makes us more fetal and more fearful. *Something in us believes that by shortening ourselves we're making a smaller target.* While such thinking may be accurate, it's not healthy. As a bodyworker and teacher I want to make you aware of this deep line muscle and challenge us all to relax and tone our psoas to make positive changes in *all* aspects of our lives.

The psoas is the deep front line of the spine; when it gets tight and tied up, the whole body suffers in some way or other. I'm not saying a tight and short psoas causes *all* the diseases and conditions we see; I am suggesting it as a contributing factor to almost any problem you have. Let's learn to release it.

Figure 5.4 shows an unhealthy psoas in the body at left. See how it shortens, tightens, moves the low back forward and spills the stomach forward and out? Notice that this unhealthy muscle also encourages the upper body *and* the hip hinge to shorten and the head to pitch forward.

In the healthy body on the right the psoas falls back, relaxes and allows the spine to lengthen and straighten out as all the hinges soften. How much easier will it be to have good posture if there's resilience, life force, vital capacity through the whole spine, but especially this area? Much easier! Tone your psoas and tone your life.

WHAT TO DO ABOUT IT

Here's my favorite exercise to encourage the psoas to learn to lengthen and fall back instead of shortening and tightening further. I don't

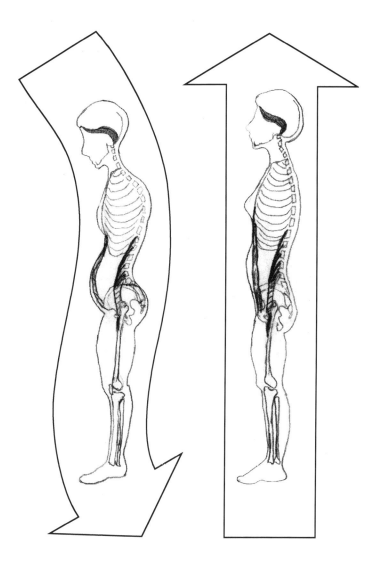

Figure 5.4 A resilient psoas relaxes into movement;
a tightened and shortened psoas must always work.
The body will lose its line

hesitate to give this exercise to any client, whether they've had back surgery or are contemplating it; whether they have a diagnosis of herniated or bulging disc or pinched nerve; even if they have trouble walking. This is a definite "do no harm" exercise that I believe does everyone good. The problem many people have with this exercise is that they can't *feel* anything happening. Sometimes they'll feel activity or awareness on the side opposite of their problem area or the leg they're moving; sometimes they feel nothing. My advice to them is "Keep at it." It's subtle but it's powerful. See what you think.

I ask clients to lie on their back on the floor. I then ask them to push/pull their low and mid back into the floor as deeply as they can. I even ask them to suck their belly button down into the floor.

The more they find this center place and tug it down toward the floor, the more this work will help them retrain and release psoas across the lumbosacral area as well as the hip hinge. Once they have the low back/belly down and back, I ask them to drag one heel and allow that knee to draw up toward the ceiling. Slowly! The slower one drags and the more one holds the stomach and back down, the more likely one is to feel the tugging of this muscle. Often, just initiating the movement, then waiting for the sensory awareness of what's happening to register, will change the way you think about psoas.

Generally I don't give clients a specific number of repetitions or times per day to do this work. I'm more likely to suggest they do it when they have a few minutes and think of it. For my style, doing two or three very slow drags with each leg, with breathing and awareness, is sufficient to condition the psoas to begin a shift that can change the

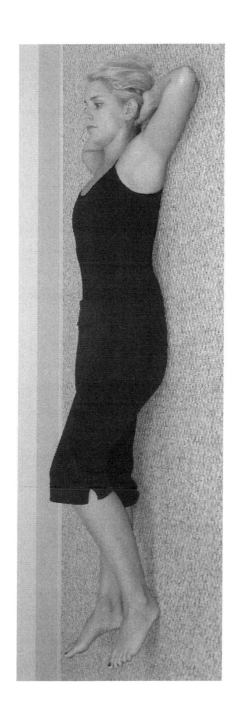

Figure 5.5 A safe and effective way to relax and release the psoas muscle

entire body, top to bottom. Once or twice a day, or when you think of it: these are the time frames I support.

Although I'd already been working as a Rolfer before my plane wreck in 1987 and had a fairly good understanding of the deep muscles of the spine, I gained a whole new viewpoint after my accident. One spinal bone was broken into small pieces. The bone exploded from the force of the crash landing; my left leg jammed into the low back and the seat belt restraint helped to shatter and disintegrate the bone, right in the area where the psoas muscle begins its journey down the spine and into the rich lumbar nerve network. Suddenly my bone was in pieces and my nerves were strangled. My neurosurgeon told me my spinal column was squeezed into about 10 percent of the space it should normally occupy. The fact that I could wiggle my toes, even though I couldn't drag my leg up or down, was a hopeful sign. The fact that I had no sensation in my pelvis or groin was not. My damage was severe and sobering.

PELVIC LIFTS AND PIGEONS

What did I do? I slowly climbed out on the wing of the plane, lay on my back, and began deep breathing exercises joined with pelvic lifts (see Figure 5.6).

I knew my back needed length. I've often wondered what would've been different if we'd landed in some remote area instead of on a busy city expressway shoulder. If I hadn't been "helped" right away, would I have been able to soothe the trauma out of my body, get up and walk away? While I believe that could have happened, we'll

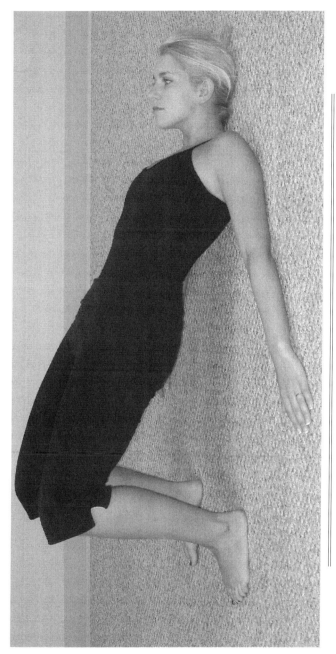

Figure 5.6 A pelvic lift is always appropriate to relax and restore the low back

never know. Worrying about choices from the past doesn't serve me in the present or the future.

I moved from the pelvic lift exercise to the earlier psoas drag. I wanted to lengthen and pull my broken tail area out of my upper spine. This was difficult, but I wanted to release the trauma so that I could heal. I was busily doing my exercises by the time the first rescuers got to the plane and "stabilized" and immobilized me. I gave up my authority and allowed them to care for me. In my painful and fearful condition, it was good to have someone else take charge of the situation.

The pelvic lift or tilt serves many of the same purposes as the drag. It also calls for length of the back side of the back. Lie on your back as shown; lift your knees and spine up toward the ceiling and out of your own low back, mid back and shoulders. Even pull your neck long. Visualize your knees and legs as one end of a hammock—let your knees be pulled toward the tree. Then let your spine come back to the ground, piece by piece, beginning at the head and working straight down the twenty-six hinges. Imagine you can pull your tail out of each of the twenty-six spinal hinges. This lengthens, straightens, removes fear and tension all up and down the spine. It soothes the psoas.

Once I was left on my own in the hospital, I decided to do what I knew how to do, and began practicing long, slow breaths which I tried to force further down into my stomach, low back, and pelvic floor. When my breath finally reached my pelvis to my satisfaction, I relaxed and slept. I believe if I hadn't had this innate intelligence that made me seek to find my breath, I might not be walking today. My lumbar nerves were screaming in fear, and had I not thought to soothe and relax them, they might've shut down altogether. It's made me curious about working with spinal cord injury victims more immediately after their trauma. I believe simple breathwork and relaxation techniques can help soothe and alleviate injuries more than we've suspected. Our inner guidance knows how to recover from our pain/fear/resistance to change; we'd reinstate breath and energy into the injury and all its holding patterns.

OH, THERE'S THE PIGEON!

Another favorite psoas stretch is called pigeon pose in yoga (Figure 5.7). Some of you may already know this pose. Go onto your hands and knees. Now, bring one knee in front of yourself and put the heel of that leg into your groin. Allow the knee that's gone forward to also move slightly outside the center line of your body. Slide your other foot long, behind you. Both knees are still on the floor, but one is forward and slightly out to the side while the other is further back with its foot stretching all the way behind your body. The back leg begins to feel a psoas stretch on the front of the spine.

With a bit of awareness you'll find how to stretch this area even further. Generally if I turn my head and upper body away from the longer, back leg I feel more stretch in the long leg psoas. I'll also try to push the longer leg's hip further into the floor. I've found that by lifting up onto the toes of the back leg, with a firm ankle hinge, I'm finding even greater territories to stretch. I'll hold this pose for several seconds and a few breaths. As with all my stretches,

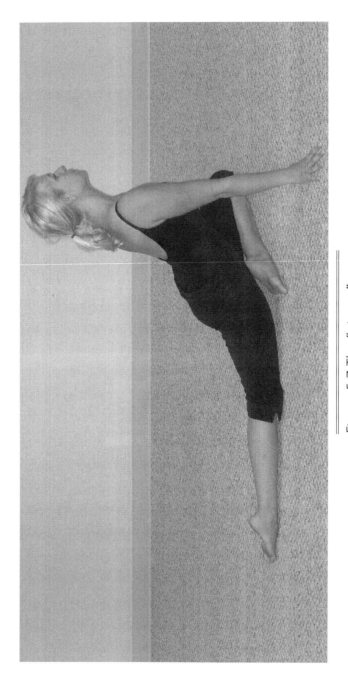

Figure 5.7 The "pigeon" pose

I'm careful not to overdo, and I'm the authority on what's right for me.

Let's add another way to open the sacred hinge and therefore stretch and tone the psoas muscle on the front of the low spine. Hang your legs over a barrier, to the knees. Perhaps you'll stretch across a couch with your knees up over one arm. Maybe you're at the landing of a stairway, or have your legs dangling in a pool. Find a place and way to allow your knees to bend while you're lying fairly flat on your back. Now…tug your lumbosacral area—even out of your tail and hip area—away from the back of your knee. Perhaps you can add an extra push with your feet creating resistance while your knees and low back stretch. Paying attention to this line can truly open the pelvic floor and bowl.

One of my students recently shared a different psoas stretch with me. She asks clients to lie face down on the bed, table or floor, and lift one foot toward the ceiling, then back toward their head. Hold this foot with your hand and draw the leg toward the head, bending the knee backwards. You'll begin to feel the stretching in the deep line on that leg and also up into the stomach and front of the back. The more you can remember to keep our upcoming stomach hinge pulled away from your sacred hinge by simply putting your stomach further back while stretching your tailbone long, the more efficiently you'll stack your spinal blocks and hinges.

Lately I've been working to open the line between hips and sacred hinge. Very simply, I lay on my back, pull the low back down, and pull or push my hips long and away from my back. Delicious!

It's my hope you'll begin to locate your deep line psoas

muscle, learn to relax and tone it, shake out the traumas you store, and have a more open life with a clear, resilient psoas. As I work, think, teach and observe, I'm truly convinced that learning to identify this muscle and its connections, learning to allow a bit of relaxation, and understanding how to keep the area relaxed are major steps on the road to finding health in your bodymindcore.

⊣ THE STOMACH HINGE ⊢

SPILLING OUR GUTS

Much of what we want to say about the stomach hinge strongly relates to the information about the psoas muscle from before. All the exercises and stretches from the previous chapter continue to make sense in relation to the stomach hinge. When the psoas gets short and tight, pulling the low back forward, the stomach and pelvic bowl are also pulled and dumped forward. The more resiliency and tone we find in the entire length of the psoas, the better our posture and the smaller our stomach. Do you see why I preach this muscle is a miracle? The more you learn to waken the psoas muscle—any part of it—the more resilient and healthy your entire body will become.

We've all seen men, some not even older, who have what we call "beer bellies". Often, I don't think their stomach is as large as they believe it is: I think their back has shortened as their stomach hinge has crept too far forward.

As we lengthen the back, soften the psoas, and create ankle and toe hinges, many of these men see a noticeable

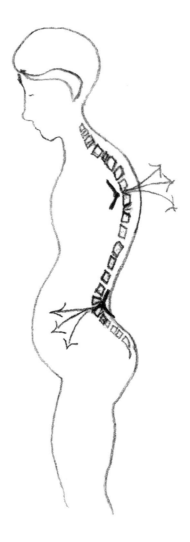

Figure 6.1 A forward stomach hinge, caused by tight psoas or other postural problems, doesn't have to be there

difference in the thickness of their waist. The same is true of women, though we see this pattern more easily in men.

TOO MANY SIT-UPS

Have you ever been a sit-up champion? That's someone who can do a hundred sit-ups in two minutes or some such impressive statistic. I think the concept of fast sit-ups can be extremely detrimental to our stomach backs. In fact, I believe my original back injury, long before my wreck, came in high school physical education class when our coach forced us to do quick repetitive sit-ups. A quick sit-up *yanks* the entire back up as a unit. Being pulled up by the external muscles *rectus abdominus* (the six-pack) on front, and the long *erector* muscles of the back, angers and creates unnecessary shortening in both these sets of muscles. And it *doesn't* create awareness in our psoas, which needs communication and exercise. I believe quick sit-ups tighten and tone the sleeve of the body *without adding energy or awareness to the deep line*, where true health resides. Reconsider sit-ups as a toning mechanism. If you use them at all, at least consider the following idea.

I ask clients to do a very few slow motion sit-ups. If they'll slowly come up in a curling pattern, vertebra by vertebra, they'll both feel and tone *all* the back muscles: Front, back, superficial, and deep. I literally encourage clients to make friends with each spinal segment, in slow motion, as they do their sit-up. As always, breathwork makes this stretch more effective. And as always, be your own final authority.

A VERY INJURED HINGE

Most of us have a short area somewhere in the middle or lower part of our spine where we can't lift ourselves in slow motion through this sit-up posture. Often it's around the stomach hinge we're discussing, or the heart hinge of the next chapter. What to do? First, simply keep trying. Often, some part of your brain will finally remember how to bring your body through the weak or tight spot. Sometimes if you'll simply anchor your feet under a couch or other furniture to stabilize them, that'll give you the extra boost you need to lift yourself through the weakness. You might want to ask a friend or partner to help you by holding your hands to slightly lift your upper body as you work through your stuck spot, giving you a tiny boost when you hit your non-firing section of spinal muscles. As you allow them to help you lower yourself back to the floor, you'll really feel the area you've been ignoring. If no one's around to help, try wrapping a belt, a rope, or a stretching strap to a doorknob or a piece of sturdy furniture.

I'd also like you to consider holding your stomach into your back as a meditative activity. What would life be like if we learned to hold our belly button toward the back wall of our spine? Make it a game. There's no losing, so let yourself win a bit.

Stand, and ask your hips and genitals to creep farther forward while your stomach back lifts and pulls straight back. Go ahead and bring your heart hinge up and forward too (working ahead!). Now, you may as well go ahead and lift your head and eyes toward the heights. This may open some new feelings. It's all right to allow them.

Our stomachs hold all the thoughts, feelings, and ideas we haven't processed or don't know how to release. If you remember my model that disease is the slowdown of energy, you'll agree many of us slow our energy down in the stomach area. We don't exercise our bodies in a way that encourages the release of this stuck energy, we ingest fuels that are bad for us, and we choose to retain instead of eliminate too much of what comes into our lives. No wonder our stomach hinge is clogged!

WHAT COULD LIFE LOOK LIKE?

What would life look like if our stomach hinge was free?

We'd live in joy, compassion, and wisdom. We'd learn to find happiness in every situation, no matter how troublesome it looked on the surface. We'd give thanks for *whatever* appeared in our lives, thereby calling greater good to us. We'd learn to forgive both ourselves and others in any situation and discern how to simply allow energy to flow instead of judging situations as bad or good.

We'd live in honesty and integrity. We'd be consistently who we are in *all* situations. If I'm one person to my spouse, another to my child, another to my co-workers, and another to my church family, I waste my energy trying to remember exactly *which* person I'm being at any given time with any group. Why waste energy trying to remember which persona to wear? One size fits all. My colleague Ibby calls this behavior "living in a seamless garment".

We'd admit mistakes freely and fearlessly. We could praise others without starving ourselves. Too many of us operate believing there's not enough love in the world, so we compete for love. My teacher Stacey used to say the quickest way to stop an argument from escalating is to simply say, "You may be right." We haven't admitted our wrong; we've allowed the possibility of a different "right" and the possibility that someone else's viewpoint is important and valid, too. When we stop, breathe, and listen more than we speak, things are great.

We'd learn to see common ground with everyone we meet. We all need to find a common ground of the spirit and realize that no matter what our values, we share spiritual similarities *if we make up our minds to respectfully look for them.* I was given a bumper sticker once that said "Self-righteousness—the unforgivable sin." I loved the sticker, but when I finally put it on my car it felt too self-righteous to display. It's hard to allow others to have their beliefs, their model, their values, their ideals when we think they're all wrong. It's also necessary.

We'd intend to be *loving and we'd* hold *that intention.* Holding unconditional positive regard for self and others doesn't have to look like lying down to be run over by anyone. It may even look angry and unloving to those still living in old patterns. We care enough to commit to working through problems instead of bottling up or running away from them. *Setting an intention to stay on the path to loving relationships is the most fulfilling work we can do.* We choose everything in our life—why not choose and hold onto a loving intention? You'll fall off the bicycle occasionally, but you can get up and get back on, with new skills you've learned from the fall. Keep the stomach happy!

Failing to be totally ready to absorb every new experience without fear (and frequently I do still fail), the next best act is to learn to process and discharge the stimulus/

trauma more immediately. My formula here is simple too. When a negative stimulus sticks in me (late-arriving client, car trouble, larger than expected bill, child getting into trouble, argument with spouse) I work to reframe it for myself as a learning moment: an experience I don't need to repeat, but that I've been blessed with to grow and learn and avoid an even worse circumstance, because of this early awareness and acceptance of the situation.

CLEAN THE DUMP

On our farm we kept a family "dump" at the back of our property, and my father let friends and family come and dump their trash there also. When my parents died, my sisters and I paid dearly to have someone clean out the family dump. How much simpler to have dealt with that trash as we deposited it instead of waiting fifty years to take on the task!

Many of us aren't ready to face pain or move through it. We'd rather stash it in the dump at the back of our property. I challenge us all to look more quickly and more squarely at our pain. If you're already stepping into your pain, go a bit more bravely. If you're afraid of your pain, take small first steps and praise yourself when you achieve them. If you're raising children, encourage them to look at their pain more quickly and fearlessly. Help them to decide to let go of old hurts and replace them with joy. See change as a positive experience. Even if you don't yet see the benefits, decide it's for your good, and believe your good will be revealed to you.

AND NOW, THE BODY DUMP

How do we clean up this hinge? We've already discussed stretches for psoas in the previous chapters and added new ones. Let's add to the downward dog from Chapter 3, the concept that you now bring your stomach hinge and your low back up into the air as you stretch yourself further down and forward.

Do you feel a good stretch? You've found another way to stretch the stomach back. Experiment with using different hinges up and down your spine in these stretches.

Here's one more chance to pull the stomach hinge back. Get into a hands and toes touching the ground position—much like you're doing a pushup. Now, walk like an animal—a tiger, a horse, a bear, even a giraffe (Figure 6.3).

Experiment with being different animals and imitate their gait. But remember you're most interested in keeping the stomach back tucked up. You're finding and retraining the stomach hinge, leveling the lumbosacral hinge and the pelvic bowl.

ANOTHER WAY TO KEEP IT CLEAN

I'm going to veer off the path of exercises in this chapter to talk about a new subject: Cleansing. Think about the congestion many of us carry around our middle—our spare tire, our fat; our potato chips, fast foods and diet sodas. We need to learn how to clean out the insides of our stomach back. Most of us know we eat poorly; few of us do anything about it. Soon we come to a point where

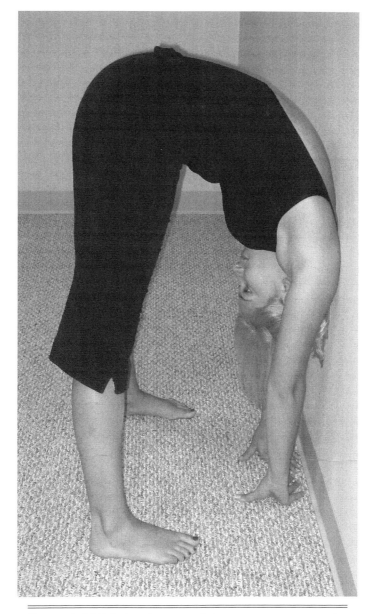

Figure 6.2 With the downward dog posture against the wall, add the stomach and back pulling toward the ceiling

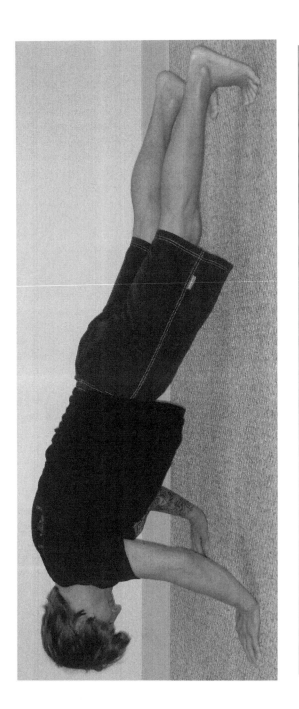

Figure 6.3 "Animal walks" while paying attention to holding the stomach back will create stomach tone and a level hinge

there's so much poison in our system we feel we must stuff in more poison to dilute the poisons already there.

Years ago I was given a tape of a nutritionist who shared a colon cleanse recipe, based on a five-day fast, ingesting only certain juices and cleansing substances. I use it about twice a year, and for me it's really effective not only to keep off excess weight; I believe it also cleans the inside of the colon, helps to keep the heart healthy, and puts less pressure on all the organs in the mid body. I'm choosing not to share this recipe in the confines of this book: I'm not a doctor and I don't want to prescribe. If you do choose to search out a colon cleanse recipe, I think you'll find many options. Most of them could help you, if you follow them faithfully and use common sense.

I've seen the worth of a colon cleanse, as have many of my clients. I've literally seen a six-foot, ropy, stringy, tar-like mess come from my colon! I've lost ten pounds easily in five days. Part of the difficulty in the process is getting through days one and two without food. The second problem many people have is remembering to come out of the fast with healthier eating habits. For several days at least, staying away from meat, cheese, dairy, and alcohol in favor of fruits, vegetables and whole grains just makes sense. Why clean out toxicity, only to add more toxicity into the body?

So, I offer this information because I know the power of cleansing the colon. Please respect it! If you'll commit to following through with the recipe you find, or are given by your doctor or nutritionist, I think it can help you make changes in your colon, your stomach hinge, and your life. But you must be serious about making the changes. As always, if you have questions or concerns, consult your physician before starting such a cleansing program.

If this section seems impossible to you, perhaps you'd be better served by going to a colon therapist. These practitioners perform colon irrigations designed to soften and remove the fecal matter that's trapped on the inside of the colon walls. I believe a cleanse/fast achieves levels of cleansing that require quite a few colonic sessions. I'm not prescribing or advocating either of these techniques. I offer the idea that if you want to open the front of the back, it's useful to clean some of the garbage away from it. Admit the gut back is responsible for carrying around an extra five to fifty pounds of fecal matter stuck inside the colon. How can your body be happy carrying such a load? How can your psoas be happy if it's trying to keep this load from falling forward?

It's my hope you'll begin to locate your deep line psoas muscle, learn to relax and tone it, shake out the traumas you store, leave your back, back, and have a more open life with a supple psoas. As I work, think, teach and observe, I'm truly convinced that learning to identify, allow relaxation, and stay relaxed in the stomach area are major steps on the road to finding health in your bodymindcore. Clean your house and live in your stomach hinge again.

CHAPTER
7

THE HEART HINGE

BREATH: OUR INSPIRATION

The heart hinge is the original body hinge I first got excited about, many years ago. I still teach a class called "The Heart Hinge" and share with students how to open this area in their clients more effectively. I'm excited to share these ideas here. In twenty-three years as a practicing body worker, and fifteen years as a teacher, I've found one of the simplest, yet most powerful ways to bring clients to health is to teach them how to breathe.

Teach them how to breathe? We all know how to breathe, or obviously we wouldn't be here. Yes, but...too many of us don't put much energy into our breath, don't bring in much oxygen, don't breathe out toxicity, and don't use this simple tool effectively. Minister and author Catherine Ponder states in her book *Open Your Mind to Prosperity* (1971, Lees Summit, MO: Unity School of Christianity, and 1984, Marina del Rey, CA: DeVorss & Co, p.103) that there is one basic problem in life: Congestion. If you remember my contention that the only dis-ease is the slowdown of energy, you'll begin to have some sense of the respect I feel for the ability to bring fresh air into the body as we clean out the waste. Too many of us are deficient in this talent—and it *is* a talent.

Look at the words "inspiration" and "expiration". Both come from the same Latin root as the word "spirit". Inspiration is the act of bringing spirit, or life force, into the body; expiration is the letting go of the spirit. Put simply, when we inspire or are inspired, we're bringing life force into the body. When we expire, the life force is no more.

Let's look also at the words "valor", "value", "valiant" and "validate"—even "Valhalla", the home of the gods. All come from a common root which encourages us to find our centered spot (is it our "vault"?) around the heart and operate from that spot.

Usually when a client comes to me for the first time, I ask them to take a deep breath, either while they're standing or once they're lying on the table. Often I see no movement at all. I wonder: Did she hear my directive? Sometimes I'll ask again: Another deep breath, please. I may see a small ghost of breath, yet sometimes nothing moves. Generally, the people who come to me breathing reasonably well have either studied yoga on a regular basis, have been singers, or have a specific reason they've learned to breathe more fully than the general public. Usually they know they breathe more deeply than others, and work to keep it that way. They understand the value of deep, cleansing breaths.

INTENTIONAL BREATHING AND
THE DIAPHRAGM

One of the ways to stay healthy in our body that we often over-look is this clean, clear, intentional breathing. It's this simple: When we remember to enhance our breathing capacity and consciously breathe more fully, not only are we creating a cleaner fuel additive for our blood and body; we also move toxicity *through* the body and *out of* it. When we don't breathe well, we starve our tissues of oxygen and allow toxins to settle into them. So the more we can learn and remember to breathe fully, the healthier we'll become.

I've often told my clients that if they'd just breathe deeper, drink their daily recommended water, and get a bit of mild exercise they'd probably never need to see me again. I don't even think they have to eat that well! Fortunately for my repeat business, too many of them don't take these instructions very seriously. But I'm frustrated, because I truly believe we could all create health in our body with these simple techniques.

The muscle I'll feature in this chapter about breathing and opening the heart is the *diaphragm.* Most singers have heard of this muscle, and some have been given wrong information about its use, I believe. First, let's look at the muscle itself.

Imagine an umbrella in your chest, which acts as floor to the heart and a ceiling for the stomach. See the edges of this umbrella as anchoring to the bottom ribs all the way around the ribcage. Imagine that in the umbrella, two funnels thrust down into the stomach area. Their function is to create a space where the *aorta* or large supplier of blood to the body, the *vena cava* or large blood return vein of the body, and some nerves flow through the umbrella.

That umbrella is the diaphragm muscle, and the two funnels are called the *hiatuses* of the diaphragm. They become tendonous as they leave the diaphragm, and

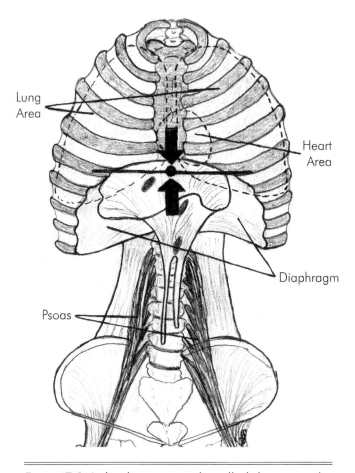

Figure 7.1 A diaphragm muscle pulled down into the stomach by poor posture will inhibit breath flow and create many other problems

eventually anchor on the front of the spine, very close to the area where the psoas muscle from the last chapter also anchors.

We begin to see how a shortened and tightened psoas muscle already tightens the breathing mechanism by pulling the heart hinge short and closed. The deep line gets constricted and breath gets squeezed. When the lungs fill with air, the diaphragm/umbrella is pushed further up with the breath. Toxic blood is pumped into and filtered through the lungs, and aerated blood is pumped out. But if the diaphragm's too tight and restricted, breath and blood flow is decreased. We lose our breath energy, we lose our blood supply in and out of lungs, and we lose our vital capacity.

If we can lengthen the front of our spine—the psoas muscle both as it travels down into the inside of the legs and at the top where fibers intersect with the diaphragm muscle—health and well-being in the entire body will very possibly follow. If we can't find a way to keep this area open, we tighten our breath, pull our chest forward, and hide our hearts. We close our heart hinge. We create both emotional unavailability and potential heart and lung problems. Let's reopen our heart hinge and expand the fetal curve we've created when we shortened the front of our bodies. Learning to breathe more effectively is a great tool to begin lengthening the front of the body.

FIBROMYALGIA

Do you know the condition fibromyalgia? It's related to chronic fatigue syndrome (CFS), and in fact, many fibromyalgia sufferers tend to be very tired *in addition* to having chronic pain throughout their bodies. Usually fibromyalgia or CFS sufferers can't get a good night's sleep, which further aggravates their condition. While some prescription drugs may help, generally, after a diagnosis these people are left to their own devices. Perhaps they'll be given a prescription for sleep as well as for pain; often these drugs only help minimally.

I believe *fibromyalgia is simply the disease of having had the wind knocked out of one's sails,* and of not being able to get the deep breath that resets the breathing mechanism. The body's stuck in trauma mode and doesn't know how to return to neutral. By this definition *we all have fibromyalgia to some degree—show me someone who's never had the wind knocked out of their sails, and I'll show you a very young or very sheltered person!* Generally the people who most suffer from this condition will confirm that physical, mental or emotional trauma took their breath away—a divorce, car wreck, financial setback, loss of a child, hard pregnancy, hysterectomy or Caesarian section surgery are common causes. Nearly always, a new client can pinpoint for me exactly what their trauma was and when it entered their body. It's my job to help them release the trauma, with the breath.

Fibromyalgia sufferers generally tend to internalize and hold onto mental and emotional tension. Often they're those who can go and go and do and do—the busy people. They keep going, through the pain and the tension, but they hurt more and more as they wind themselves tighter and tighter. It's important for them to learn to breathe out the old hurts, traumas, and toxins that they've stored and left unprocessed in their bodymind. Often I'm able to help fibromyalgia sufferers simply by getting them to remember how to breathe, and then suggesting they look at relaxing their own attitudes toward how much they must achieve in their lives. All of us will profit by remembering this as we allow breath to flow into and through our hearts.

If fibromyalgia was a wind-knocked-out-of-my-sails disease of the 1990s decade, I believe our new epidemic disease is even simpler to describe: *We're too busy to breathe!* Too many of us have developed what I'll call "waitress mentality". If you've ever been a wait person, you'll have a sense of what I'm describing. A good food server does two or three different tasks with each trip across the dining room. Likewise, we've all taken multi-tasking to far too complicated heights. We need to simplify!

OPEN THE HINGE AND BREATHE

So, let's start our breath awareness simply. Just lie down and focus on long and deep breaths. Keep your back in the floor or bed. Use pillows if you need them. Just imagine that you take longer to bring air in and out. Learn to focus (or pretend to focus) your breath into various parts of your body: your head, neck, arms, chest, low back, tail, pelvis, and knees. It's less important to find all these places right away, and more important to experiment with longer, focused breaths. If you can only breathe in for a count of three, ask yourself to reach for a five-count in-breath. If you can achieve fifteen, try for eighteen. Expand your breath capacity.

Now, put some fulcrum under this heart hinge area. It can be as simple as a small pillow or rolled-up towel;

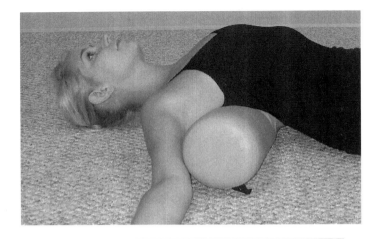

Figure 7.2 Create a bolster to further open the heart hinge

it may be a couple of tennis balls, or potatoes, or a shoe. Find the spot that seems shortened on the front of the body, place your tool underneath, and focus on expanding breath as you're opening this stuck hinge.

I often work over an arm of a couch: lying on my back, first my head goes over the arm and tries to open up my neck hinges by bending the head backwards. Then I move a bit further down the spine, trying to open up the "dowager hump" area, where the head pulls forward, at around C7/T1. I'll keep working down the spine until I find the tightest, most shortened piece of spine, usually right at the heart area. The idea is to coax the spinal hinge that's too tightly closed and ask it to open and stretch. Then, breathe! Let breath energy flow through the front of the spine again. Visualize the psoas and diaphragm muscles letting go of each other and lengthening the front of the body.

Another good exercise, both for this section of the back and a later one as well, is the yoga posture called the cobra. This is a simple (not easy!) posture where you lie face down on the floor and begin a pushup, while allowing your stomach and low back to continue to try to stay on the ground.

The more you arch the upper body, the more you open the heart hinge. As always, breath is still an important part of what you're doing. Take a deep breath, stretch the front of your spine as long and curved open as you can make it. Relax, and then try again.

And a classic favorite exercise is a simple backward bend. If we look at the posture of a computer worker, we'll see how easy it is to continue to shorten the front line of

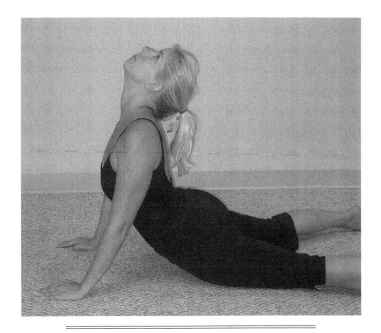

Figure 7.3 The "cobra" position from yoga

the body. We know we've gotten into "achievement mode" and we need to remember to open things up again. I find simple backward bends are helpful. Stand, or stay seated if you want. Allow yourself to gently stretch as far backward as you can. Remember, breathe!

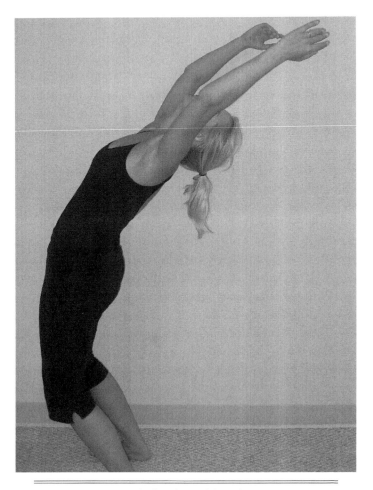

Figure 7.4 A simple backward bend can open many hinges, including the heart

This isn't about you working so hard that you fall over backward; it's about you learning to bend over backward in a way that stretches and opens the entire front of the spine, plus the heart hinge and the diaphragm area. You'll remember that in earlier chapters we've spent time bending forward; it makes sense that we need this back bend as a counter-balancing movement.

Have you tried exercise balls? There's really an art and science to choosing the proper balls for your body, your needs, your size. If you've never worked with balls, experiment with laying over various sized ones, on your back. Can you feel new areas opening in the heart territory? Even though this chapter is about the specific heart hinge, experiment with moving more energy into every hinge of the spine in turn, clear from the head hinge and down through the sacred and hip hinges.

A separate new tool we're finding available through more fitness suppliers is a foam roller. These range in sizes, but many are about eight inches thick in a cylinder. You can use them all over your body to give yourself a good workout. This section of the back is a particularly good place to use such a roller.

RULE OF THIRTY TIMES SIX

Here's a way to enhance your breath capacity and to release pain and holding from your body. I call it my "Rule of Thirty Times Six". First, know that thirty is a goal, not a given. Lie on the floor or bed and get comfortable. Pay attention to slow breathing. We're going to set a goal that you can train yourself to breathe in for a count of thirty seconds. Eventually we'll also try to breathe out for a count of thirty seconds. In between the breath in and the breath out, we'll add a quick exhale/inhale before expelling. Remember thirty is a goal! You may not be able to go much past four or five when you first try intentional breathwork. Don't worry about failing; just keep trying to lengthen your count. Imagine you can slow down the intake or exhale stream of breath. This will help you take longer. When you reach the point where you think you can't inhale more, try to hold that breath, then take a couple of shallow sniffs in for another two, three or even five seconds.

At the end of such an inbreath, two things will probably happen. First, you'll need to quickly expel when you've stayed at the top of your breath for so long. But just before that happens, pay attention to your chest. You'll probably feel tension through your chest you didn't even know was there. With this breathwork you'll begin to acknowledge and release tension through every in- and out-breath. It's both at the top of the inhale *and* the bottom of the exhale that you'll feel changes in your body. So stay on the edges of your breath! You'll begin to feel places you hadn't acknowledged for a long time.

During this Rule of Thirty Times Six, inhale very slowly and incrementally; then quickly move through the out/in so that you can concentrate on a slow exhale. *I concentrate on completing six thirties in and six thirties out:* thirty in/quick exhale and inhale/thirty out/quick inhale and exhale: repeat this pattern six times. *The number thirty is totally arbitrary:* you may find your best breath only reaches fifteen. That's all right; just keep stretching yourself to breathe a bit longer. You may be able to go to sixty. Think how much oxygen you're exchanging, how deeply you're cleaning the tissues and enriching the blood through your body! I always take myself to the top or bottom of my capacity; then I try to gulp or expel just that last bit more. That's how to stretch the breath.

In addition to bodywork directly at this psoas/diaphragm connection, I believe in the importance of teaching a client how to monitor their own heart hinge area. This may be as simple as changing posture when sitting at the computer or desk: Why do we always bend forward from the same one or two hinges only? Why does our head creep so far forward when we work at the computer, causing our heads, necks and shoulders to be painful? Why couldn't we use different hinges in our spine? What about people who drive a lot, or fly frequently? Can you see how a car or airplane seat also encourages us to shorten this heart hinge area?

A client movement cue I sometimes use has occasionally caused a client to burst into tears when they hear it: "This week, lead with your heart as you go forward."

And have I mentioned lately that you need to remember to breathe?

Pay attention to how you're breathing, and see a full breath as an extension of how happy you are to be part of the world. Many of us close off our heart hinges to make a smaller target for the slings and arrows that come at us daily. *If you can enhance your breathing capacity, you can enhance your capacity for enjoying the world. And if you decide to be happier in your world, I think you'll find you're breathing easier.* I don't care from which direction you decide to make that change, but I challenge you to make it. I believe letting breath flow through you will allow you to drop old coping patterns and find out who you want to become in the present.

CHAPTER 8

THE ARM HINGE

ONE ARM, MANY HINGES

It intrigues me how, the longer I ponder the concept of hinges in the body, the more I see each hinge as having attributes that create its functional and structural uniqueness. The arm hinge is such a place. This hinge is one of the most complicated places we'll examine.

Very simply stated, I believe if one tries to reach out and do good works, to *serve*, with tight arms and a tight neck, one can't enjoy their service. Conversely, if one is serving at work they don't enjoy, their arms and neck will tighten. Pain and congestion will result. What's the bottom line? *Find work you love and do it joyfully. At the least, find how to make your work more enjoyable and devote energy to staying relaxed and free in your body as you work.* We'll talk more about learning to give with open arms later in the chapter.

Most simply, the mechanism of this arm hinge is at T1, the first thoracic vertebra. This is the area of the spine at the base of the neck where one bone is usually more prominent. It's often referred to as the "dowager's hump" area, because as we grow older and our head pulls forward even farther, this hump increases. It's this dowager's hump area from where our arms grow and are innervated and supplied with blood. All the work we do in the next chapter with hinges down the arms will be based on the idea of first keeping this arm hinge open and clean.

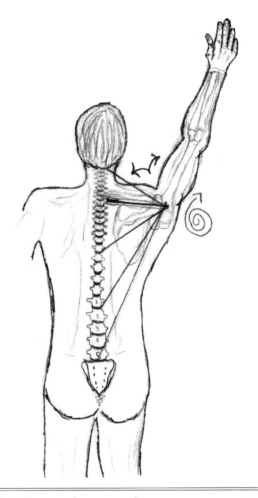

Figure 8.1 The arm hinge can be seen as originating at the neck (occiput), the dowager hump (C7, as shown), the tail (lumbosacral junction) or any hinge between

A NEW TYPE OF STRUCTURE

One of the unique features of this hinge for me is that it shrinks and expands somewhat like an accordion. That is to say, it can be one inch of hinged material or thirty inches up and down the spine. When we're reaching above our heads with arms, the hinge is not just at T1; it might reach all the way down into the middle or low back. Yet, if we're keeping our arms low to the ground, for example stooping to lift a heavy load, our arm hinge may reach up into the back of our neck. It will move up and down the spine depending on what functions the arms are performing.

A second factor that makes this hinge different is an additional connector of the arm to the body. The collar bone or *clavicle* joins the arm to the *sternum* or breastbone at the front of the body. *This is the only place where your hand, arm and shoulder are attached to your body by a bone.* The clavicle's therefore something of a stabilizer or strut: the spinal bones form the hinge, but the collarbone helps hold the hinge in place.

It could be argued that the arm begins at the back of the head in the brain back. Follow the *trapezius* muscle, which looks like a diamond from the back of the head, out to the shoulders and down to the middle of the back between the shoulder blades.

If the neck is too tight the trapezius will shorten and tighten, pulling the shoulders and arms up into the ears. Many of us go through life in this state.

But what if we raise our arms over our heads? Now the line of pull is from lower down our back, and we could say our arms grow out of our tailbone. As we raise our arms,

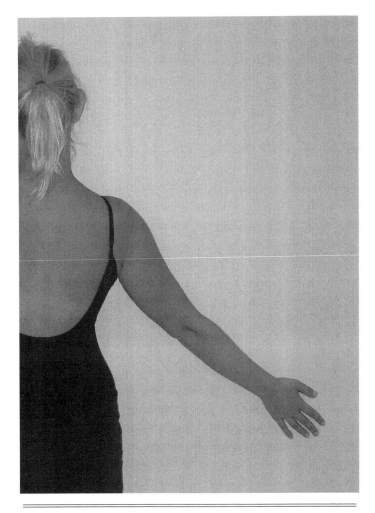

Figure 8.2 An arm hinge beginning at the head and neck

we can begin to feel this pull from the lower part of the trapezius.

And there's another muscle called *latissimus dorsi*, or widest of the back, which starts all the way down at the tailbone, travels up the back and out toward the shoulder,

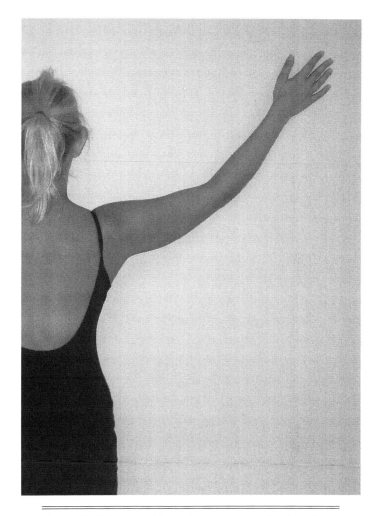

Figure 8.3 An arm hinge beginning in the low back

and anchors on the backside of the arm at the back of
the armpit. As you think of this muscle and trapezius, you
begin to see how both anchor the arms into the lower
back. Imagine a hairdresser, a barber, a bartender who
stands with arms forward, and anchors the weight of the

arms and their activity into their low back. Visualize a computer operator activating the muscles from neck to arms. Depending on the direction in which the arm travels, a different section of the back can be activated and taxed.

The arms are an important part of our overall machinery, that which differentiates us from many other animals. With arms and hands we reach out and perform tasks: writing, driving, painting, massaging, cooking, sanding, gardening, fine crafting—the list of things we can do as a result of having arms and hands that aren't just used to move us across the earth is astounding! And as our backs get tightened, anywhere, the arm line must shorten and hinder the way our arms work for us.

It's not only bodyworkers and massagers who have problems keeping arms free. I see people from all walks of life who've injured themselves by tightening and over-working their arms and shoulders all the way into their backs. It's only *if and when* we get these clients to realize they need to reexamine the way they work their bodies that we can help them get better and freer for the long term. To restate: No one can work hard, tighten their body, force it into work mode, and not suffer. And when one is doing joyful work, one is much more likely to stay relaxed.

ATTITUDE IS EVERYTHING: WHAT'S JOY LOOK LIKE?

Many self-help books have been written with titles that let you know over-achieving isn't what you really want to do with your life. All of us want to succeed; too many of us believe suffering is necessary to bring about success.

Suffering is optional! It just takes some time for us to learn to shift our attitudes toward achievement into attitudes of gratitude and satisfaction with what has been accomplished instead of shame about what hasn't yet been completed, perfectly.

So, having first made this plea for you to realize how your attitude toward your work is important to how long your body will last, now let's proceed to the techniques we're examining to unwind the arm back as yet another form of decongestion of the body. In this chapter we're trying to pull the arms out of the back—either the upper, the lower, the middle, or all. You may have a sense of which direction you need more, based on how you usually use your arms; but I'll also suggest to you that pulling your arms out from any direction won't hurt you, and will probably help you.

HOW TO UNWIND

I've thought about this at length. I don't believe stretching an area is necessarily better than tightening an area of the body in order to open and relax it. It makes sense to me that change in either direction is change, and change is good. So I like the feel of stretch, length, and looseness that comes with a good stretch. But sometimes I get as much or more relaxation by simply tightening an area as hard as I can—my neck, my low and mid back, my shoulder, my sacroiliac junction. Sometimes I'll try to shorten and tighten and feel my bodymindcore reach an internal realization: "Good! That's tight enough. Now, everybody can relax a bit, since we've finally found tight enough." When my back hurts from standing or sitting too long, I find the tension, then simply tighten/hold/release, tighten/hold/release and I feel a deep relaxation everywhere.

When I've worked long and hard, I often grab one arm just below the elbow with the other hand and simply pull—I try to pull my arm out of my shoulder and my shoulder out of my neck where I feel the tension of the arm hinge. I pull to a place where I feel the stretch but not to where I hurt myself. Then I put breath into the stretch. Often I can release an amazing amount of tension just by a good tug on each arm. I also like to simply reach my arm up into the air and stretch. If you've ever watched a cat really stretch, you know something of what I'm suggesting. Cats are able to take one leg and pull it to a great length, often while stretching their low back and tail in the opposite direction. So this idea is simply, pull your arm out of your back, stretch, and breathe.

To make this stretch even more effective I often pull my head to the other side. Try this: Touch your ear away from the stretching arm into your shoulder as you pull one elbow away from your body. Do you feel how you're adding another dimension?

I've long wondered if more people have problems in their necks coming from their shoulders, or problems in their shoulders coming from their necks. I've finally decided the answer is "yes", and it doesn't make any difference which way you chase it. If someone is having neck issues, they have shoulder issues, and vice versa. If we can unwind one area, we unwind both places.

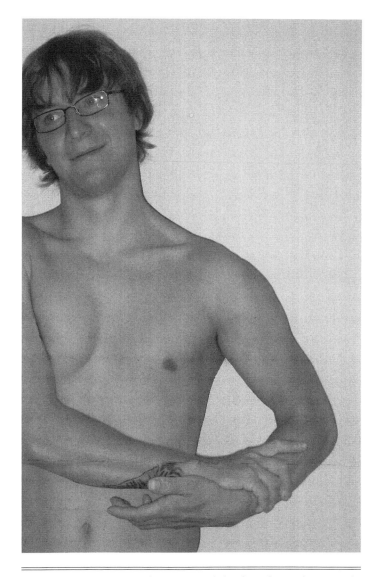

Figure 8.4 Engaging the arm and the head simultaneously creates a greater stretch

DR. ROLF'S ARM ROTATIONS

Ida Rolf left very few exercises that she suggested were life-changing. The arm rotations I'm going to describe are one of two that I know. Here's how she tells us to open our arms: Lie on the floor on your back, knees up. Put your arms out to the sides at shoulder height, as far from shoulders as you can get them, with palms down into the floor.

Now stretching the arms out to the sides, lift them up toward the ceiling and toward each other so that they make a half circle from the ground toward the sky. Bring

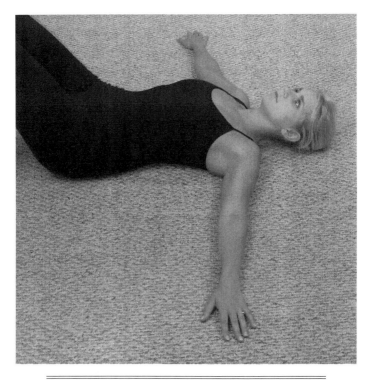

Figure 8.5 Dr. Rolf's arm rotations, position one

your hands together as you reach for the ceiling in a way that allows the backs of your hands to try and touch each other.

Your shoulders don't need to leave the ground, even though you're trying to lift and stretch the arms. Bring the arms back down to the floor, palms still facing down into the floor.

Now, for step two, rotate the arms, *from the shoulders, and if possible from all the way to the spine,* one quarter turn, so that your thumbs now reach for the ceiling and try to touch each other. Again bring your arms up to join each other; then bring them back down. In step three again

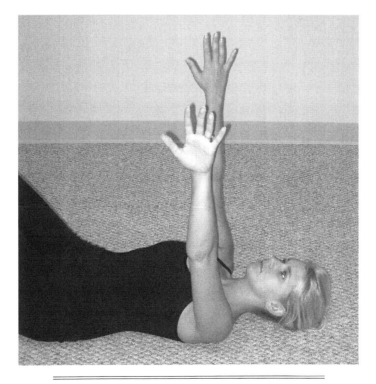

Figure 8.6 Arm rotations at the top of step one

you rotate from the shoulders. The palms are facing up toward the ceiling before you bring the arms up to touch the palms of the hands together. Bring them back down, and step four is one more rotation, so the little finger now points toward the ceiling.

As you finish this stretch, you've been through four steps. Repeat step four; then bring the arms down to the floor again, but now de-rotate the arms from the wrists *while still pulling them out of the shoulders*, so that the palms are again facing up. Take the arms through step three, back down, and de-rotate at the wrists again so that thumbs are pointing up. Backwards through step two, back down, and de-rotate so that palms are again facing down. Do this last step, stop and relax.

Did you feel how each time you moved through the stretch you found a slightly different path for the arms to follow, with a slightly different stretch of the muscles of your arms and shoulders? And if you really understood how to de-rotate the arms from the wrists instead of the shoulders, you found another new set of muscles as you reversed the steps. I find this to be a great stretch to do whenever I have a few minutes and have been in a particularly challenging task that involves arms. Whether it's painting with a roller, massaging, driving long distances, cutting hair, working at a computer—any of these tasks can benefit from a relaxation brought on by arm rotations.

OTHER STRETCHES

An easy way to open my shoulder girdles and arms: I find a counter, a stairway railing, or a surface about waist height

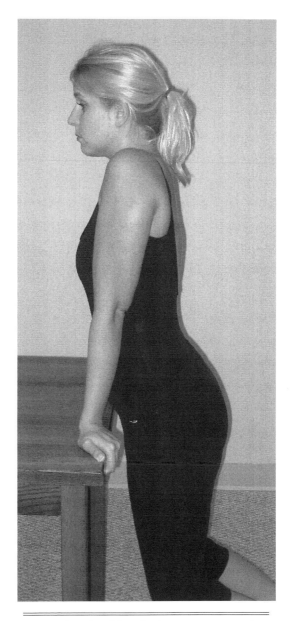

Figure 8.7 A table, desk or counter makes a good piece of exercise equipment

that will hold my weight. Then I place my hands on the stationary surface and lift my body weight up off my feet as far as I can go; allowing my spine to try to shake loose and lengthen and stretch all its segments.

I can stretch my lumbosacral and hip hinges out of my arm hinges. When I get into this position, I'll sometimes hear and feel the various vertebrae break loose from each other, and when I come back to a standing position I'll also feel taller and freer all the way through my spine and also through my arms. Changing hand position and direction will give you different stretches, too. And if I must, I can even use this stretch while sitting at my desk, by placing my *elbows* on the table. Sink your weight into them; then pull the stomach hinge back while settling longer into the lumbodorsal hinge. Again, how many hinges can you open or shake out as you work down the body?

Another favorite stretch is to simply put my fingertips on a doorframe and hang my body weight off the fingertips. Obviously I can't always put my entire body weight on the door trim; I might pull it off. I gauge how well the trim will hold me, and how much weight I'm able to put on the frame.

I'll breathe while I stretch and try to feel the lengthening all the way down to my tailbone. Some days I'll stop with the idea of just hanging off the frame; other times I'll try to begin a pull-up to fire up and stretch the muscles of the arms. If you're shorter you may need a step stool.

Many of us didn't have good training in our high school physical education class. We were taught to quickly pull and jerk ourselves up instead of paying attention, going slowly and working through the entire line of fingers, wrist, elbow, shoulder and back hinges when we did

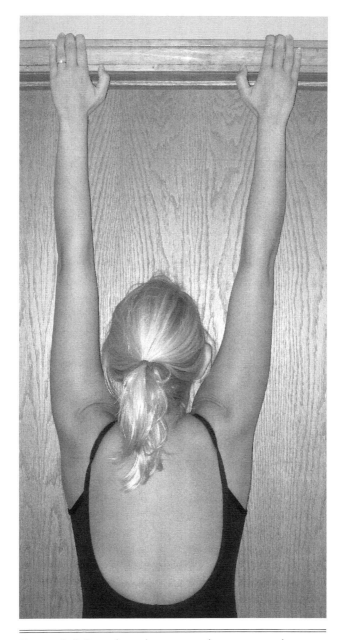

Figure 8.8 Stretching lower arm hinges in a doorway

the pull-up. So when I hang from the doorway, or try to pull myself up toward it, I work to enjoy the sensation of muscles firing that have been on "rest" mode for too long. When I'm hanging, I think I'm stretching *and* tightening the low back; when I pull-up I think I'm talking more to the neck branch of the arm back.

All of us overuse our arms. All of us overwork on at least some of our tasks. A bit of attention to keeping the arms open will make our lives happier. A bit of attention to pulling the arms out of the back, the neck and the heart can add years to both our effectiveness when we're on task, and to our lives. Coax your arms out of your bodymind-core, take a breath, get out of achievement mode, and go out into the world to serve with joy!

SHOULDERS, ELBOWS, WRISTS, AND FINGERS

FRONT LEGS FROM THE SHOULDER AND DOWN

While it could be argued that each of the above-named hinges deserves its own chapter, we're going to talk to all four at once. I've become much better at releasing arms since I began treating them as front legs. Whether you believe in the evolutionary change of man coming from four-legged status into two-legged isn't important to me; I do know the similarities between arms and legs have made it easier for me to do good work on the arms. Similarities are: both limbs have one large bone in the closer segment (thigh and upper arm), both have two bones with a membrane between in the lower segment (leg and forearm). There are arches in hands and feet, many moveable hinges in fingers and toes, and a ball and socket joint where arms and legs join the main body. As I work either limb I achieve more when I keep similar principles in mind for both.

But, since we no longer (if we ever did) see these "front legs" as weight-bearing limbs, things have changed. Since we seldom put weight through the wrists the way we put weight through the ankles, wrists have lost importance in terms of weight-bearing even as they've gained importance in terms of their ability to carry out detailed movements that differentiate us from other mammalian beings.

Let's start with the shoulder hinge. Here we have a ball and socket (actually called a "saddle") hinged joint, much like the hip socket.

However, the hip joint is far more difficult to dislocate because the socket of the hip is larger and more difficult

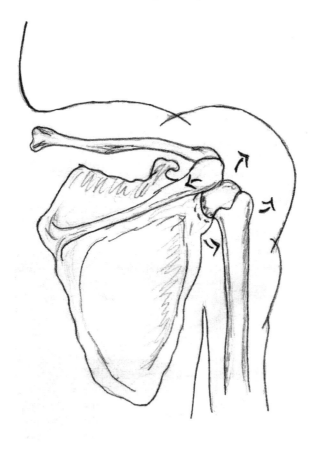

Figure 9.1 Like the hip joint, the shoulder moves like a ball and socket hinge

to exit, and because there's more tendonous tissue that anchors the hip together. The shoulder roams much more freely. Again, isn't this in part because we don't expect to put weight into it as much of the time?

The next hinge, the elbow, can easily compare to a knee hinge in many aspects: it has the same fairly horizontal hinge action with a bit of wavering or sideways movement in the track of the hinge.

What's the back side of the knee is the inside of the elbow; they move on different planes, but their function is very similar, moving on a straight track.

And while the wrists likewise only rarely bear our weight, some of the exercises we're going to attempt in this chapter will hopefully let you see a great correlation between the functions of wrist and ankle hinges.

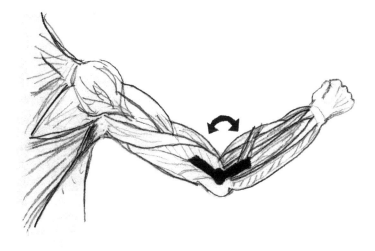

Figure 9.2 Flexion and extension of the elbow can easily be compared to similar movement in the knee

If a healthy ankle moves fluids through the lower body and into the upper, wrist hinge health probably assists in returning fluids through the upper body. Simply learning to bend the wrists back, put a bit of weight into them, and encourage a stretch can be almost as powerful to the

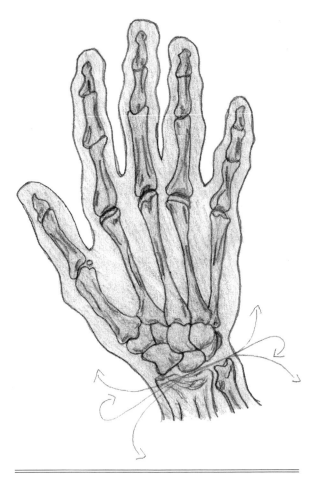

Figure 9.3 Like an ankle, the wrist can find many directions in addition to its back and forth track

bodymindcore as learning to develop the ankle hinge of the foot that too many of us have forgotten.

We'll add finger hinges into our chapter both to equate with the toe hinges and because much of our day-to-day work has created problems in our arms all the way to our fingers.

Think of some of the tasks we perform: writing, computing and mousing, detail work; many of the tasks we perform require us (we believe) to carry a great amount of

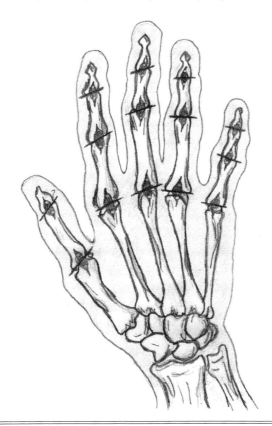

Figure 9.4 Fingers (carpal bones) and toes (tarsal bones)
operate in a similar fashion

tension in our finger hinges. This tension will translate and travel all the way up into the elbow and shoulder, into the arm hinge, and beyond through the entire spine.

What can we do to keep these four hinges free? We can start with any of the exercises back in the previous chapter. Any work from that chapter *must* begin to release tension through the arm *simply because it's releasing tension at the root of the arm, at the arm hinge in the spine. As we open the deepest point of connection of the fingers to the center of the body, the fingers begin to open also.*

THE CORE* PHILOSOPHY
(*COAX ORDER, RESTORE EASE)

In my CORE Philosophy, each of us is a six pointed star—the head, tail, arms and legs are the six points. I like to encourage clients to realize each of these six "superficial" or "sleeve" points has a deep line.

The deep line of the arm goes all the way both up to the back of the neck and down to the heart, the gut and the low back. When you begin to realize the fleshy pad between your thumb and first finger is the terminal point of that deep line you can start to stretch and unwind in a totally new way.

So, hanging from the doorway trim as in the previous chapter, doing mild pull-ups, placing your weight on a counter or table and raising yourself; all these stretches for the arm hinge are all clearly stretching the shoulder hinge also. Depending on the angles and positions you find to put your hands and elbows into, you'll find you can stretch them also with these stretches.

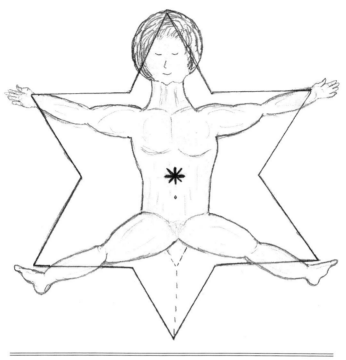

Figure 9.5 When we're tight at the CORE, the points of our star aren't free to express and lengthen

PUSHING IT UP AND OUT

One of my favorite stretches for all the various hinges through the arms is the old-fashioned modified pushup position with knees in the ground. I'm less interested in making all my weight be lifted up and down through my arms; I'm more interested in challenging all the hinges of the arm. I'll keep my knees on the floor, lift myself through my arms, and try to feel the stress or tugging in my shoulders, in my elbows, and in my wrists. I find if I allow my elbows to bend to the outside I really oil that hinge; yet if

I focus on hanging from my shoulders I have an entirely different experience. If I also sink into my wrists while I bend my elbows, a new sensation of stretching arises.

Sometimes I'll also use this pushup position from my elbows—that is, I'll rest my upper body weight on my elbows as I try to lift my upper body. I feel a different stretch in my shoulders and arm hinges. Experimenting both with elbow pushups and with changing the position of the wrists and hands, when you're working in pushup position, will again show you different lines of tension you're holding onto in your body. Remember to pay attention to the entire spine, even when you're stretching the shoulders.

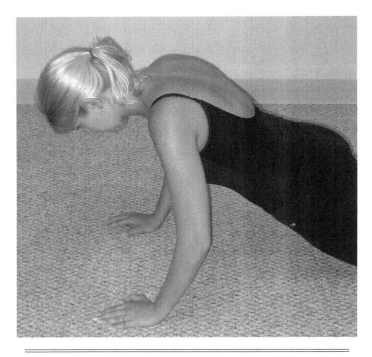

Figure 9.6 Working the arms with "meditative" pushups

Remember the "animal walks" from the stomach chapter? Let's revisit them. This time, in addition to remembering to lift your stomach hinge into your back as you walk, let's also think about stretching out the lumbosacral hinge, and really working to feel each of the hinges out of the arm— the shoulder, the elbow, the wrist, and the fingers. Work them all, allow energy to flow through them. Remember to try walking like different animals—a turtle, a horse, a dog, a lizard. Imitate walks to find new muscle groups.

WHAT'S CARPAL TUNNEL?

Let's get specifically into carpal tunnel pain. This choking of the carpal or wrist tunnel is often a repetitive motion injury—factory work or some task which entails a monotonous repetitive job, and usually with the above achievement mode for speed factored in also. First I try to teach my clients to breathe and relax while they're working. This is extremely hard for someone who's on a factory line and processing one unit every three seconds in the same motion all day. But sometimes a client can self-correct with this simple work. It's an earlier question come back: How does one find breath, joy and relaxation while staying on task?

I invite carpal tunnel sufferers to relax all the way into their neck and their arm back, breathing and stretching. Then I ask them to lie on the floor, put their hands over their head; then to put their palms flat on the floor above their head with arms bent backward.

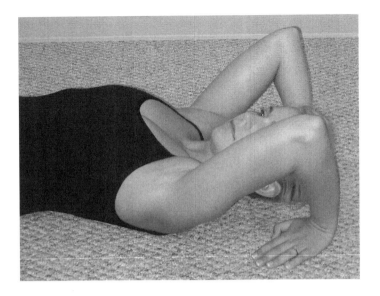

Figure 9.7 A simple release for carpal tunnel pain

I want the palms down into the floor, elbows toward the ceiling and the fingers pointing toward the shoulders and head—the arms are curled up into themselves. Then I suggest the client begin a pushup of sorts—trying to get the fingers and wrists to stretch into a new pattern from where they've been working.

When I stay in this position and try to apply a bit more pressure to the finger and wrist hinges, I believe I'm draining much of the tension I've created in my hands. As always, remembering to breathe as I work this stretch gives me a more effective stretch. It's my belief that we generally shorten and tighten the flexor line of the arm with the work we're doing in the factory; and that by opening the line backwards we'll begin to stretch the muscles we haven't been using—the muscles that have been putting the brakes on for the flexors.

Is there any real need to go surgically into the wrist and cut tissue in the carpal tunnel, when just learning to stretch the tendons will almost always cure the problem?

Another simple stretch for the finger hinges: Stretch an arm out in front of you, bend the hand back so the palm is facing away from you and the fingers point toward the ceiling.

Next, grab one finger tip and simply pull it back toward your head. Allow each finger to be stretched in this manner; then all of them at once. You'll feel stretches and tensions in the fingers connecting to pains in your arms which you didn't know you had.

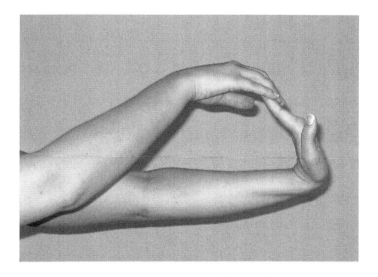

Figure 9.8 When was the last time you stretched your fingers?

STRETCHING THE "GREAT ELIMINATOR"

The fleshy point where the thumb and first finger join is called in acupuncture circles "the great eliminator". I've heard at various times that stimulating and squeezing this point can alleviate headaches, stop seasickness, assist the liver in dumping toxicities, aid digestion, and even induce labor in a pregnant woman. I personally know it's a powerful point to change the hands, elbows, shoulders, arms, and further; all the way to the heart. I'll often grab this point for myself on both front and back of the thumb pad, then simply squeeze and try to breathe deeply as I milk the point. This simple squeeze helps us to not only open the deep line, but also to pull the fingers out of the shoulders.

RULES TO LIVE BY

I've long been impressed by Dr. Jerome Frank's book, *Persuasion and Healing* (1961, Baltimore, MD and London: The Johns Hopkins University Press) written mainly for his own psychiatric community. I resonate with his idea that *illness is present because people are* demoralized, *and that to heal them, we need to "re-morale-ize" them* (my word). We need to help them find and stay on a purpose that gives them joy and juice in their lives.

In his book Frank suggests four conditions must be successfully met before a person can be healed. First, the client must believe their practitioner truly cares about them. Second, the setting must be appropriate. To me these first two points suggest that if a client feels comfortable, safe, and trusts their practitioner, they've come a long way toward health.

Third, the practitioner must communicate his or her healing model. They must explain their system, what it is, what it does, and how it can work to heal the client. If the client can hear and understand what's being done and why it should help, and it makes sense to them, they're set to receive healing. And fourth, the client must be an active participant. This can be as simple as asking a massage client to drink more water; it can be as complex as asking a client to severely change diet, or perform movements during a bodywork session, or break a pattern of entering destructive relationships. Only when a client's invested in the model and committed to doing the work will they truly get well. Isn't this a fascinating thought?

Aren't these good rules to live by, no matter what our task? I think this model serves us in every aspect of our lives. Ponder the concept of living on purpose: You'd care about your work, you'd create a positive setting, you'd be passionate about explaining what your work is, and you'd enjoy bringing others into your passion. And you'd have enthusiasm and joy in your life.

LOVING ALL OF SELF, ALL THE TIME

Carl Jung added the term "shadow" to the therapeutic vocabulary. I understand the shadow as those parts of our personality that we've rejected, masked, or buried because of our own fears, ignorance, shame or some other lack of love moving through us. *If we made a list of all the parts of ourselves we didn't like, then worked to find the gifts and the positive sides to these shadow parts, we'd integrate into our bodymindcore in yet another way.* If we didn't possess a quality, we wouldn't see it in another; conversely, what we see in another is a reflection of what we see or are afraid to see in ourselves.

Part of the shadow experience is listing all the reasons we can't do or be that which we'd like. Only after we acknowledge our inner objections, fears, and barriers and allow them to speak to us, will we be able to clearly see our path ahead. When we overcome those resistances and simply take that leap of faith, amazing things can happen in our world.

How do I serve? First, by deciding how to find passion in my current work, or finding a work for which I have passion. There's a story of a man coming to the wall of a new town and asking the gatekeeper, "What are people like here?" The gatekeeper asked, "What are they like where you come from?" The man answered, "Dishonest, un-friendly, stingy liars." The gatekeeper answered, "They're like that here. Come on in." When a second man came to the gate and asked the same question, the gatekeeper again asked, "What are they like where you come from?" The second man answered, "Salt of the earth, best people ever. They'd do anything to help you." The gatekeeper answered, "They're like that here. Come on in."

AS WE THINK, SO WE ARE

It really is that simple. Our perception shapes our world. If you believe you're stuck in a dead-end job where no one appreciates your service, it will be true. Yet if you believe that your job, no matter how small or insignificant it seems, is a vital cog in the machinery of the Universe you'll find satisfaction, perform well, be noticed, and find that the next step is a step to a higher level of responsibility and fulfillment. Find the passion.

Years ago I was given a quote from one of the Rolf instructors, Ron McComb. I'd like to share it here:

> Today, I'm able to put into words a discovery arising out of a long held suspicion that there is a strong connection between the hands and the core through the emotions. That is, that the hands are an extension of the ego. The hands protect the core and give it nourishment. That forearms become tight from continually defending the core against perceived threats to the ego/body, whereas open forearms and hands are disconnected from the ego and therefore become connected to, or are, an extension of the heart...such as in the hands of the Buddha. That is, instead of moving compulsively from the ego, the hands wait to be moved by the heart.

I believe the deep line I'm so interested in freeing surely runs from the heart, out the arms, and into the hands. Put into emotional terms: When our heart's in our work, our hands are willing. If our hands aren't about the work we want to perform, our heart is hardened and unhappy. Where are you?

THE HEAD HINGE

A DOUBLE HINGE

As we've worked through the body, it seems nearly every hinge has an aspect or two that makes it different from every other: the ankle looking like an axle allowing the hinge to rise or fall from side to side; the hip in its ball and socket; the lumbosacrum holding the entire spine in balance; the shoulder much like a hip ball and socket with a clavicle support bone. Each hinge has a different personality. The head hinge is no exception.

The way I'm going to describe the head hinge is something like a tri-fold screen where hinges can fold back in either direction. See the front of the throat as one of these hinges, and the back of the head where it joins the neck as the other hinge.

Can you reason that if one pulls tight, the other suffers? And conversely, if one finds length, both are opened?

"HEAD UP, WAIST BACK"

Ida Rolf used to tell clients that even if they didn't have time to get bodywork, they could say to themselves when

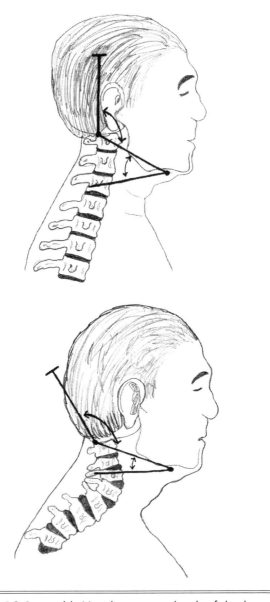

Figure 10.1a and b Head up, waist back: if the head
hinge is seen as two hinges pulling in different directions,
one sees the complexity

they think of it, "top of the head up, back of the waist, back." This isn't as easy to do as it sounds. Generally when I share this idea with clients, they lift their head and pull their shoulders back, and are quite satisfied until I point out that, to do so, they've just shortened, tightened and pulled their low back forward. As soon as clients try to relax the low back and place it where it belongs, the head chooses to move forward again. Often it takes several tries before they understand the feeling of keeping the head long and back while the back stays back and knees bend slightly. Once they find the spot we're after, however, they want to hold onto it. They feel taller and more in charge of their world. How could that be a bad thing?

It's true. When we stand tall, we feel tall. Gravity can't weigh us down because we're balanced around a central beam or line. But if our heads live out in front of our bodies, our necks work hard to keep them from falling forward. An eight to twelve pound head can end up exerting about fifty pounds of pressure on the neck muscles. They try valiantly to keep it from toppling off the body, but think of the stress they endure in this job.

We've got to learn to get our heads on straight, not only so that we're less depressed, but also so that we don't have to work so hard just to move through life. The payoff for getting the head tall is the creation of yet another open section of back, all the way to the brain!

HOW DID WE LOSE IT?

Imagine a girl of twelve who has grown six inches in the past year, before any of her friends find their growth.

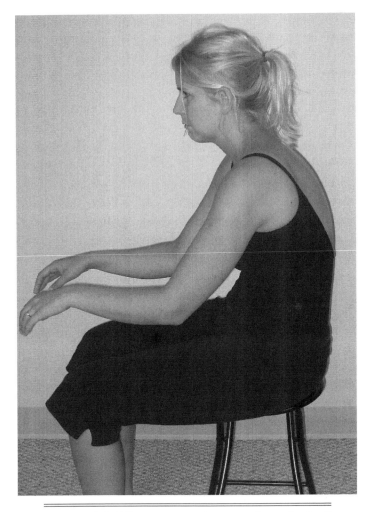

Figure 10.2 When we stand or sit tall, we feel tall

Think of a girl who realizes she's the only girl in her class with breasts. We all know how important it is to blend in, to not be seen as different; because we've all had at least a small case of low self-esteem. What will these girls do? Probably the easiest solution such a child can find will be stooping forward, shortening the front deep line of the body, and trying to take up less space. Why can't we teach such a child to claim that space and become the goddess she is, instead of encouraging her to hide her light?

Think of a young man sitting at the computer for hours at a time—either as part of his job, or because he just loves the connectedness—his personal favorite addiction. Realize how, when he stands after hours of holding his head in front of his body, it feels wrong to find his head up on top of his body. It's impossible to get your head on straight when you spend most of your energy training it to live far in front of you, and that's what much of our world teaches us to do.

I remember the psalm, "I will lift mine eyes to the hills, from whence cometh my help." It hints to me that as far back as Old Testament times, we've had clues we need to learn to hold our heads up, back, long, and regal. Lifting the eyes while lengthening the back of the neck will change a person. It's that simple. It's not that easy.

Often when I work with clients to lengthen the head hinges I'll suggest to them:

> Think of a general. He sits at the top of the hill and watches the overall battle take place. He's never worried for his personal safety, and he feels totally supported by his staff. Now, think of the foot soldier down on the front line. He sticks his neck out and gets his head blown off. Which would you rather be?

I encourage them to visualize their head as the general, being carried around by supportive shoulders.

Clients often respond well to this image and lift their head off their chest and back into the air where it belongs.

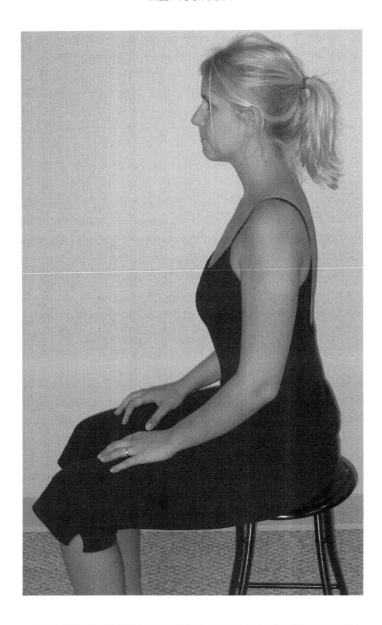

Figure 10.3 A straight posture invites energy to flow to and through the head hinges

SHORT AND TIGHT

Too many of us have tension in the jaw and tongue—
working to find and relax the area on the front of the neck
may be a new concept, but one I hope you'll consider.
Think of the people you know who have TMJ (*temporo-
mandibular* joint) problems—tightness of the jaw muscles
that make people grind their teeth at night, or give them
incredible headaches. Perhaps you're one of these people.
Does it make sense to you that some of the tension in your
jaw, or their jaw, may be about things they'd like to say;
but they've chosen to "bite their tongue" instead? Can you
believe that if a person learns to express their "negative"
emotions more freely, there will be less tension stored in
their jaw, tongue, and neck? And do you see how tension
in the jaw can translate to headaches up behind the ears,
jaw pain, stiff shoulders, and even difficulty swallowing?

Even more simply—just take a moment to thrust your
own head forward in front of your body. Can you feel the
tension created by this thrust?

Can you feel a spot at the base of the skull tighten and
pinch? That pinching is your brain stem being deprived of
energy. Pull the top of your head both up and back. Can
you feel a loosening of the brain stem area? The area of the
brain known as the stem, the root or tail of the brain, has
also been called the "animal brain." It's the oldest part of
our brain, and takes care of basic survival skills. The newer
brain may make plans; the older brain simply survives.

When the back of the neck gets short and tight the
survival brain is choked. The *occiput* bone at the base of
the skull gets pulled down into the neck. The *atlas*, the
first cervical spinal bone, wedges forward between occiput

and the *axis,* or second cervical bone. The spinal column is pinched, and the liquid flowing through the spinal column, the *cerebrospinal fluid,* is no longer able to flow freely.

Suddenly because of tension at the brain stem, the river of nerve impulses is congested. Open the brain stem by taking away the threat to survival, and the entire body is nurtured by that energy flow. The twelve *cranial nerves,* which control all the sensory functions in the head— smell, taste, hearing, etc.—no longer get choked. Release congestion, restore circulation.

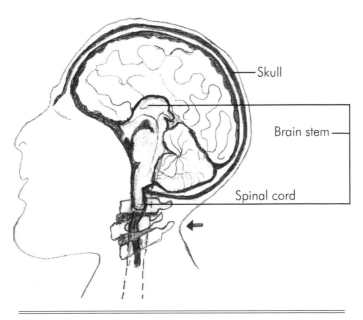

Skull

Brain stem

Spinal cord

Figure 10.4 When the head hinges shorten and tighten, energy is diverted from the head

What about those of us prone to headaches, especially migraines? Does it make sense that there's too much tension in the head hinge, and that if we could begin to loosen the tension, energy could again flow and headaches could be relieved?

DEEP HEAD LINE: LOOK TO THE HILLS

What's to be done for people who live with tension in their head, neck, shoulders, and jaw? The first action is, literally, to teach them to get their head on straight. Ida Rolf gave us the idea, and it's a great beginning to simply start by working to check your posture. Realize that we've chosen to pull the front line of our body short, bringing the head forward and down, and we stay in that position. Simply being aware is a great first step in changing and opening that line. After practicing keeping the head up and back for a while, it becomes a less strange and uncomfortable place. Eventually, you may find you don't want to go back to the old standing and sitting postures.

Experiment with closing your eyes, putting your head up and back as we've just tried, then *lifting your eyes*—looking toward the ceiling. Remember to keep the back of your head long as you raise your eyes at the same time, and to breathe. Do you imagine you feel an opening deep inside your head?

TRACTION

Here's a simple technique you can use for yourself to try to open up the *occipital* area—the base of your skull where it joins your neck. Prepare a tool. It may be as simple as a

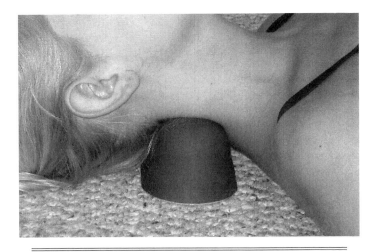

Figure 10.5 Find or create a tool to help you lengthen your head hinge

rolled-up towel. You could also put two tennis balls into a nylon stocking and tie it off to create a fulcrum under your neck. Lie on your back on the floor.

Slip your "tool" behind your head at your brain back. Lengthen the back of your neck so that you feel a tugging in this area. Pull the back of your head long and your chin to your chest. Allow your low back to tug both long toward your feet as well as down into the floor. Stretch and breathe. As you breathe, you may notice that the tension slows or shortens your breath. Tug everything a little less. Coax your breath to come up into the back of your head. See the breath reaching up into your neck, head, and brain. Open the restriction in your spinal column!

If you have a trusted partner, ask them to use a terry cloth bathrobe belt, or a rolled-up towel, and place it at the brain back (Figure 10.8). Have them give a mild tug as you breathe. If you can't get a breath, guess what? They need to lighten up. Talk them into creating the right amount of pressure so that you feel the tug, yet are able to breathe deeply without overworking. A little pressure is good, but too much is still too much.

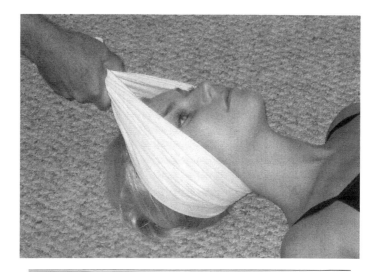

Figure 10.6 Mild traction given by a trusted partner will help to unwind tight head hinges

Perhaps when you grew up, you were taught to imagine you were suspended from a string. This was meant to improve posture, and the intention was very close to what I try to create for clients. I've found it effective to suggest they have *two* strings attached, however. One is hooked at the base of the skull, the head hinge; the other is just below the breastbone on the front of the body, the heart hinge. Do you see how opening and lifting from both these places will absolutely lengthen the head and create the length we want? And if you try to do this with regularity, you'll see why I say it's not an easy awareness until it is.

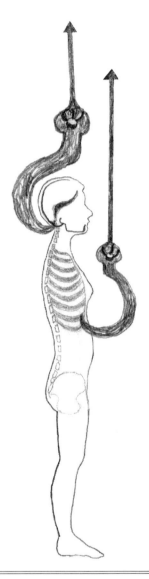

Figure 10.7 Imagine two hooks
lifting you toward the sky:
one at the sternum on the front,
one at the occiput on the back

REMEMBER TO GO THE OTHER WAY

As you'll remember from earlier chapters, I'm a fan of backward-bending postures. Too often we remember to forward bend. We sometimes forget to "go the other way". I've previously mentioned the pigeon pose and the cobra. As you opened your front line in earlier chapters, you already noticed a greater opening of the heart hinge. Now, practice finding the head hinge. Remember how I called this hinge two separate hinges joined together? As you lengthen the front of your neck, then tuck your head forward and keep the back of your head back, you'll begin to understand what I'm trying to teach you.

During my Rolf work and CORE Bodywork I also work inside clients' jaws in later sessions of my series. My intention is to loosen connective tissue that holds the jaw too tight, but my technique is based on keeping the client present and relaxed all through the deep line. While I'm working, I'm asking them to breathe, relax, allow tension to filter away, and learn to let go of the deep line, all the way up and down. Many clients learn to do this work for themselves.

Try this: Lie on your back. Now, pull your head hinge long, as if someone was trying to pull your head out of your spine. Feel that length and remember to breathe and relax into it. Keeping the tension of a long neck, raise your tongue to the roof of your mouth, then, actually begin to stretch it back down into your own throat. Remember to keep the neck both long and back into the floor or table, even focus on keeping your legs and inner arches soft and open. Create as much length as you can, then stretch the tongue also. You may even feel this stretch go into your

— MEET YOUR BODY —

low stomach! As I'm working in the jaw, clients often do feel this deep stretch into the belly.

NECK ROLLS

We've all seen, or been, the person who loves to roll his or her neck and make delicious cracking sounds, which seem to free up a rusted neck hinge. I think this isn't a bad idea *unless* one gets fixated and releases only one hinge consistently. Then it becomes hyper-mobile while hinges above and below get even *less* movement. I've begun asking if we could oil all twenty-six hinges in the spine, pretending each is the only hinge that moves the neck around.

Pretend you can roll your neck *only* right where it joins the head. Lift your head as long and tall as you can; then simply draw circles in each direction with your head, *while keeping your lower neck immobile.* This isn't easy, but the more you isolate this specific upper hinge, the more you put energy into your brains! And once you've isolated this one hinge, work on down the spine, trying to roll and relax each specific spinal hinge. And remember how we tried to backbend every hinge in turn during stretches in Chapter 7? Let's work all those same hinges, but: twist and roll in every direction you can invent. We now see flexion/extension to front and back, side to side, and a rolling, twisting motion in every segment of the spine.

"ACHIEVEMENT MODE"

Let's go back to the question of how this tension developed in the jaw and neck area. As we've said, many people have job-related neck and jaw tension, exacerbated and enhanced by their inability to remember to breathe into and through their upper bodies while they work. They're in "achievement mode", instead of "relaxed process." Perhaps sexual abuse closed their jaws and throats. And there are those people who'd rather "bite their tongue" than make waves. Occasionally I find a client who's been choked by an abuser, further shutting down the throat. Sometimes something as innocuous as poor dental work is causing tremendous jaw problems. I may ask questions to try to identify the seeds of this tension, but it's more important to help clients remember to stay tension-free as they get on with their lives.

Too many of us are still stuck in old traumas around the head, neck and jaw; we can't keep our heads on straight. We've regressed into survival mode. Learning to let go of this old pattern may be the beginning of unwinding and realigning the bodymindcore. Is this old pattern still serving us? What can we do to shift it, and how can we stay ahead of the old pattern if and when it tries to come back? When we ask these questions with intention to learn and change, we're truly getting our head on straight.

AFTERWORD
PUTTING THE HINGES ALL TOGETHER

INTEGRITY

When Ida Rolf created the work which has come to be known as Rolfing, she far preferred the term "Structural Integration". The words "integration", "integrity" and "integrate" seemed magic to her. This is what every session of bodywork should hope to achieve. So let's take a few minutes to integrate the ideas from the previous chapters and let you take them away in your own understanding.

First, allow yourself to see all the hinges of the body and realize you've often shortened or tightened or closed off your own hinges. All the stretching you've done with this book has encouraged you to remember how to open them again. In my view, we could all be taller, if we'd simply stretch all the hinges longer to stand and sit straighter and taller. It's that simple.

STRETCH YOUR HINGES
AWAY FROM EACH OTHER

For all the stretches we've created through the book, I'd like to leave you with one more challenge: How can you create stretches from any hinge to every other hinge? How can you pull the toe hinges from the arm hinge? The sacred hinge from the hip hinge? The heart hinge from the head hinge? The elbow hinge from the stomach hinge? I see this challenge as a never-ending process. I've been pursuing it for many years, very consciously for the past several. I see it as a magical journey of reclaiming my body and my space. I hope it intrigues you and keeps you working to find the new spaces inside yourself too.

I'm returning once more to both this concept of stretching hinges away from each other, and to Ida Rolf's contention that pain is resistance to change. I think many of us are happier staying in our pain because we're afraid to climb out of the box we've put ourselves into. We don't want to make changes in our lives. As painful as our circumstances are, we believe we have some understanding and control of them. When we consciously look at our patterns, we're challenged to change. Too many of us don't want that to happen. We'll complain, but we'll stay in our old ruts instead of making the effort to climb out of them. If you've made it this far in the book, congratulations! Clearly you're interested in changes in your world as you get to know your body.

WHY ARE YOU HERE?

Why are you on the planet at this time? What's the special talent, the special gift, that you have and no one else can express in quite the same way? Are you a soulful singer? A nurturing parent? A gifted writer? Do you have the ability to see both sides in an argument and help the parties find agreement? Do you have the gift of discernment, to immediately understand the bottom line in a question while others bog down in the details? Can you persuade others when you feel passionate about a subject? What's your spirit's special gift or talent, and are you using it to the fullest?

Many books have been written on the subject of finding your soul's purpose. Many tell us to find something we love to do, and the Universe will reward us; we just need to find a purpose to find happiness. The fields of pop psychology and self-help are filled to overflowing with books to tell you how to live a fuller, better, happier, more prosperous life. There's probably not much I can add to the literature already printed. But I've put my thoughts together in my own special way, so I feel I'm on purpose. I believe I'm sharing what I offer in a way that can help people live happier and more fulfilled lives. That's a noble purpose, and I'm grateful I've found it.

I'm a believer in gratitude, and am grateful that I remember to live in it. I truly believe that whatever the Lord of my being looks like, s/he doesn't want or need my praise and worship, but s/he truly enjoys my gratitude. When I focus on staying in gratitude, more good things happen to me. The old truth is still true: "Unto him who has it will be given; to him who has not, it will be taken away." Learn to live in gratitude!

It's a good feeling, that being on purpose and grateful. It helps one to get up early in the morning with an enthusiasm for the day. It helps one to go to bed with a feeling of accomplishment. It helps one remember gratitude all through the day, for that which is happening in one's life. When we're on purpose, life is lived enthusiastically. When we lose our purpose, life is endured.

If you could do anything in the world that you wanted, knowing that money wasn't a consideration because of your unlimited wealth, what would you do? Would you rescue animals? Would you shelter unloved children? Would you work to save the planet? Would you feed and clothe the sick and needy? Would you decide to focus on making more money? Would you work for yourself, or quit working? Would you be with your current partner, or your current friends, or would you create new relationships? Would you live where you live, or would you find a new spot and start again? What would you do if money wasn't your determining factor in decisions? What would you change?

Why aren't you doing these things?

DO WHAT YOU LOVE

We can always find reasons why we're not doing the things we'd love or want to do. Perhaps we feel trapped. We have the spouse, the kids, the job, the mortgage. It's not so easy to just pick up and move to Mexico to save sea turtles. *Then, here's a big one—what will people think?* What will they say? We need the approval of others that tells us we're living the life they want us to live. That approval is often far more important to us than actually living the life we want. *Further, what's the use?* I'm only one small person. I can't make all those changes by myself. I can't save the turtles, or the rainforest, or the starving children. It's too big a job for me. That's a job for someone with *power!*

WHAT'S THE USE?

Remember the story of a little boy, walking down the beach to pick up starfish and throw them back into the water? In the story, a man comes by and asks the boy what he's doing. He says, "I'm throwing these starfish back into the water so they can stay alive." The man points out to the boy that there are thousands of starfish washed up on the beach every day; he'll never be able to get them all back into the water, so he may as well give up because he can't possibly make any difference. As the boy picks up another starfish and throws it back into the sea, he responds to the man, "It made a difference to that one."

WHAT WILL PEOPLE THINK?

The second reason I cited above for not doing that which feeds your soul is "What will people think?" My short answer to that question is, "Who cares?" I've given up on the idea of pleasing people around me, and as a result I seem to please them more. It's not my intention to displease anyone, but it is my intention to be that seamless person I mentioned earlier. I want to be the same person for my wife, my daughter, my minister, my co-workers, my students, my clients, friends and family. If I'm true to myself more and more of the time, those around me come to both expect and appreciate this genuineness. *If I share with friends and family just how important discovering my soul's purpose is, but they persist in telling me why I can't attain my goals, I'll just have to stop sharing my goals with them.* As Jesus said, "Why are you casting your pearls before swine?"

I'M TRAPPED!

This belief is a difficult one. Sometimes, we really do feel trapped, and don't know how to free ourselves. What do we do if we really want to go off and study whales in Antarctica, but we have a spouse and three children who depend on us for sustenance? We can't allow the children to starve, and we can't allow the spouse to accept the entire responsibility for raising children we've chosen to bring into the world. What do we do?

And the answer to this question is, we do what we can. Perhaps you're not ready to move to Antarctica while your children are still in the house. Does that stop you from reading everything you can on the whales you want to study? Does it mean you can't make a vacation trip or a work trip to see the area you've dreamed of? Does it stop you from saving or collecting money to save whales, or to finance a trip that may be years away? Does it prevent you from dreaming who you'll be if and when your circumstances change? Does it prevent you from taking the small steps toward your goal that you're able to take right now?

HOW DO I SERVE?

Do you see how we make our own choices? *How do we serve? By creating a world where we believe in the possibilities instead of the problems. We serve by listening to our inner knowing, and finding those behaviors and people who make us feel vital, alive, and on purpose.*

There are many variations on a simple theme that's

seen in the Bible, in much of the self-help field, in the current best-sellers, and in the common sense of people who pay attention to their world. This theme is simply put: "What you focus on expands." If you focus on how tired and miserable you are, it will be more so. If you focus on how happy and wealthy and grateful you are, it will be more so. If you focus on the way you want to spend your time and see yourself creating ways to make your time more like your visions, it will be more so. *When you know what or who it is you want to be,* focus on the feeling *of the condition you want,* and give thanks *for everything that is, your blessings will be added to you.* When you focus on the feeling of being trapped in your world and your body, you will be more trapped.

As I close this book, I want you to know how honored I feel that you've shared time with me, and that you made a commitment to yourself to unwind and love more of yourself. As long as you're striving to know yourself better, you're serving the world too. I offer my blessings and my unconditional regard to you; I salute you for your good work. Meet your body; oil your hinges, find your joy, live your life fully.

Noah Karrasch may be contacted at www.noahkarrasch.com

INDEX

Printed in Great Britain
by Amazon.co.uk, Ltd.,
Marston Gate.